ACCEPTING DISABILITY

ACCEPTING DISABILITY

Hoyt Anderson

Disabled Resource Services
Sacramento, California USA

First Printing, 1994

Library of Congress in Publication Data LC Catalog Card Number 93-73180

ISBN: 0-937743-01-1

Published by: **Disabled Resource Services**
P.O. Box 163656
Sacramento, CA 95816

This book is dedicated to those who live with physical limitations and are struggling to maintain dignity and self-worth.

Acknowledgment

I wish to thank my mother, Lucille B. Anderson, who assisted me in the preparation of the manuscript.

I wish to thank Richard Treadgold who gave me the first insight and encouragement to publish this book.

I wish to thank Robert H. Schuller for his inspiration and possibility thinking messages. Many of the quotations highlighted in the boxes, are not my own, but were first spoken by him.

Desktop Publishing by:
Vito D'Albora, Sacramento, CA

Table of Contents

Acknowledgments

Preface

Preface

Today, there are approximately 12,000,000 disabled adults living in the United States, along with about 600,000 physically impaired children. Some were born with a birth defect, while others were injured later in life.

No matter the reason for the impairment, life for these individuals is never easy. For instance, one young woman whose boyfriend shot her near the brain, must sit in her wheelchair or lie in bed, not able to move any of her limbs. Although she has a keen mind, she is unable to speak. Often she becomes angry and depressed, as she gazes out the window with a forlorned look on her face.

It is quite understandable why such a person would be angry or depressed in such a circumstance. For certain, few of us can truly understand, what it is like to live with such severe impairments daily. <u>The emotional impact such a disability has on one's life cannot and should not be underestimated.</u>

However, in such a circumstance there are just two alternatives. **Life has only two options.** The one you choose will determine the quality of your life no matter if you are twenty-six or ninety-six. These approaches to your circumstances are available to all of us each minute of everyday.

Some people when faced with health impairments often surrender to their circumstances. They are quick to become bitter, critical, and feel they have been dealt a bad hand in the poker game of life. Such a person is prone to sit back, wallow in self-pity, and expect others to give them a free ride through life. They view themselves as losers, bemoaning their situation, while not trying, or not expecting much for themselves.

But there are another group of individuals who have made a different choice. They are determined to cope rather than mope, reach out rather than look back, and dream rather than vegetate. Such a person sets goals, generates enthusiasm, and determined to lead a happy productive life despite their disability.

Now, which group are you in? Do you want to live a zest-filled life? Do you want to succeed in areas you never thought possible? **Then this book is for you.** You don't have to be manipulated by outside forces, but you can learn to row your own boat to greater success.

The purpose of this book is to help you chart your own course over the rocky sea of life. **You Can** surmount most any obstacle you face. I have used at one time or another most of the principles in this book. Like many of us with physical impairments, there are times of discouragement. But I have bounce-back ability. So can you! It is my sincere hope that this book will provide constructive guidance and inspiration for all those who read it.

Hoyt Anderson

Chapter 1

Why Go On?

"You will never walk again," Dr. Water, the attending physician, told Shelly as he leaned over her bed with tears in his eyes. "Your spinal cord was severed in the automobile accident."

"Oh no doctor," screamed Shelly. "Please tell me its not true." I have been a cheerleader now I'm a cripple. I want to die." She burst into tears.

After hearing this news, she had constant thoughts of suicide. For a long time after her release from the hospital, Shelly would lie in bed without any motivation, wishing she was dead.

For some people, accepting their disability is difficult—taking weeks, months, years, or even a life time. Not only are individuals become sad, some develop anger and jealousy. This was the circumstance with William Peters, an eight year old who had cerebral palsy. He had an awkward gait, slurred speech, and an inability to walk long distances. William, and his able-bodied brother Mark, both belonged to the Cub Scouts.

As part of their activities, the Scouts planned hikes into the foothills. Mark always went along on these outings, but the leader told Mrs. Peters that William would be excused because of his handicaps. During the weeks prior to the trip, William would become hostile towards Mark and treated him disrespectly. On one occasion William shouted to Mark, "Why can't I be like you? Some people get all the breaks. If you are ever hurt and can't walk, you will know how I feel. I hope you have that experience!"

Each time Mark heard his brother make such statements, he felt unhappy because he loved William and wished they could be together on the hikes. However, despite the counseling of his parents, teachers and social workers, William persisted in displaying rage and envy toward those not disabled.

Besides rage and envy, someone disabled may experience a profound sense of guilt, particularly if that person was once healthy and strong, but due now must live with some impairments. This was true with thirteen-year old Bonny Homes.

OneFourth of July, she and her mother stopped at a fireworks stand and purchased some Cherry Bombs. They were given a list of safety instructions and were told to read them carefully. Upon returning home, Bonny was eager to light the bombs and continued asking for them. "OK,OK, I will allow you to do it yourself," Mrs. Homes replied after Bonny had nagged her for an hour. "But read the instructions first. Be careful, and make certain you are back far enough to avoid the possibility of injury."

Without listening closely to the warnings, Bonny took the fireworks and went outside. She lit the fuse but did not stand a safe distance away, and suddenly the bomb exploded in her face. Seeing this, Mrs. Homes called an ambulance and then came running to the aid of her daughter. Bonny was taken to the hospital, where she had to undergo skin grafts resulting from the accident. The intensity of the blast left Bonny permanently blinded in both eyes.

After her release from the hospital, Bonnie stayed in her room or moped aimlessly around the house, grasping the walls to feel where she was going. Bonny could not accept the fact she had lost her sight. With continuing feelings of deep regret, she recalled the Fourth of July and her mother's caution about the danger.

"Mother, if only I had paid attention to you. If only I had been more careful, I would be able to see now. Why, Mother? Why? Why didn't I listen to you? I'm paying the price by living in a sightless hell. I feel so guilty. How can I forgive myself?"

The previous illustrations demonstrate how some individuals react negatively to living with a disability. It's not easy. From personal experience, I know the torment of physical pain and the despair.

Emotional Well-Being

Probably one of the best reasons for dealing positively with your condition is to have good mental health. Many disabled people go through life experiencing self-pity, depression, anger, or guilt that interferes with peace of mind. Don Roberts, who has cerebral palsy, attended a special school for the handicapped until he was twelve. Then Don was placed in a classroom with non-handicapped peers. Soon after, he began having prolonged periods of anxiety which were accompanied by suicidal thoughts. Over the next twenty-five years he was in and out of mental institutions, made countless visits to psychiatrists, and took heavy dosages of tranquilizing medications. After much treatment, Don realized that he had low self-esteem, and with regular counseling sessions, Don is accepting his physical limitations.

This is not uncommon, some disadvantaged people have a poor appraisal of themselves. There are many reasons for this. Let's look at three of them. First, the individual may be experiencing feelings of self pity and simply viewing his condition with despair instead of focusing on personal assets. Secondly, parents or family members relate to the impaired with an "I will take care of you" or "my poor crippled son or daughter," attitude and thus in effect are saying that due to the person's injuries, he or she cannot be a productive member of society. Third, friends, strangers, and others who come in contact may react negatively to the individual, giving the impression of rejection. Of course, all these precepts are faulty since Dr. Karl B. Carlson, a physician born with cerebral palsy, in his autobiography, <u>Born That Way</u> states, "Every human life has a purpose, and even the most handicapped can be useful to society." Everyone needs to remember this statement and focus on it during moments of hopelessness.

Mental Alertness

Negative emotions can be so intense as to cloud the mind and impair alertness. This has many adverse effects, such as jeopardizing one's safety.

Billy, a sixth-grade student who walked with a limp, was going home from school. While strolling along, he kept thinking how some of his classmates had mimicked his gait during lunch period. He seethed with anger, and kept thinking, "Why was I born with an awkward gait? Why must I be the object of scorn?"

Without realizing it, this young student wandered into the middle of the road. Suddenly, there was a honking of a car horn as the driver, leaning out of the window, called, "Get out of the road. Do you want to get killed"? Luckily, the auto had stopped quick enough to avoid hitting him, but his emotions had placed him in danger. He could have been severely injured. If Billy had just ignored the remarks of his peers and not allowed himself to become agitated, he would not have had negative thoughts causing him to lose control of his better judgement and to react poorly in this situation.

Keep Hope Alive

So

You Can Survive

Physical Abilities

Sometimes an individual's unwillingness to deal with his or her limitations can have a detrimental effect on the person's physical condition. Emotional disturbances can impair bodily functioning. While this can be true for those without handicaps, in certain cases, the disabled who experience nervous reactions, find them more of a hindrance. For instance, this was quite apparent when Bob Smith, a teenager with a speech impediment became distressed during a conversation with his instructor after class.

At the beginning of the year, Bob had enrolled in a driver's education program, hoping he could learn to operate an automobile. During a conversation with his teacher, Mr. Baker, a few weeks later, Bob received some disappointing news. "I don't think you will be able to obtain a license. You do not have good enough control," Mr. Baker told Bob. With tightened face muscles, Bob mumbled, "Oh, I must drive. Isn't there any possibility I can learn?"
After learning he would be unable to drive, Bob became so distraught. He was unable to speak well and his speech became incomprehensible.

Depending on the nature of anyone's impairments, some emotional conditions can affect them physically. This is particularly true of many people with cerebral palsy. In certain situations, especially those involving spasticity, adverse psychological states of mind such as fear, anger, guilt, or depression can increase muscle tension and lack of control. Consequently, when people with physical limitations experience an inability to control their emotions, it can affect physical performance.

Social Acceptance

Acceptance of a disability allows a person to interact better with family, peers or friends in the community. Not many people will respect others over a long period of time who consistently complain and pity themselves. Likewise, anyone who appears angry, having viewed his or her state as an injustice, or envies an able-bodied person, can find difficulty gaining social acceptance. This was the case with Harry Williams, who was paralyzed from the neck down.

After almost a year in the hospital, Harry was ready to leave but did not want to go. He believed his handicaps, made him worthless. After returning home, Harry stayed in his room all day, not wanting to do anything for himself. His mother often talked with him, attempting to convince her son to develop a more optimistic attitude toward life, but her words were not heeded.
Harry became increasingly dependent on his family, While feeling that they treated him fairly. He lost respect for others. Daily, he screamed from his room, "I want to die. I want to kill myself." Finally, one afternoon Mrs. Williams became so disturbed with Harry's behavior, she phoned Mr. Thompson who was his social worker.

"My husband and I can't keep our son any longer," she lamented. "He just stays in bed, threatens suicide, has no motivation, and constantly expresses displeasure with everything we do. He is disrupting the family and I feel Harry should be institutionalized."

Mr. Thompson came to the house, lifted Harry into the car, and took him to a local hospital where he was placed in a psychiatric ward for treatment.

Harry made life so miserable for his parents that they could not cope with his behavior any longer. This situation illustrates how negative attitudes and low self-esteem contribute to lonliness and isolation.

Educational And Vocational Rehabilitation

Disabled people with low self-esteem can hamper their educational and vocational training. They think handicaps prevent them from making progress and have the mistaken idea that they are unable to learn certain skills. This was true of Bob Jones, a mildly retarded eighteen-year-old, who was enrolled in a training program to learn zip coding for possible employment in a post office.

Following Bob's graduation from high school, a counselor from the Department of Rehabilitation made an assessment of his skills, and determined that he could learn to sort mail. Bob was sent to a local workshop for training. On the first day of Bob's enrollment, Dan Clark, an instructor, observed that Bob was uninterested and watched the others.

"Why are you not working?" Dan inquired. "Come on - get involved in the program."

"I'm not well today," Bob responded.

For the next two weeks,Bob refused to try any of the assignments or to participate in the instructional sessions. Dan finally became concerned about Bob's behavior.

"You must become more active and attempt to try what is taught," Dan said in a firm, but friendly tone of voice. "Don't you want to have the opportunity of gaining employment?"

"I can't learn," Bob snapped. "I can't...I can't...I can't...I'm handicapped."

He continued to resist taking part, and refused to put forth effort in comprehending what was taught, always using his disability as an excuse to not work.

While it is true that some disadvantaged people do have difficulty mastering new skills, professionals had closely examined Bob's skills and were certain that he could master the task. However, Bob thought because of his injuries, why try learning? In such cases as this, an individual might use his or her bodily impairments as an excuse for not trying. Many disabled people are working. Perhaps, you can. But first you must believe that it is possible.

THE ME I SEE

IS THE

ME I'LL BE

Physical Independence and Self-Care

The degree to which a person becomes physically independent and responsible for one's daily needs, requires a positive appraisal of his or her capabilities and a strong determination. Today, there is much emphasis on assisting disabled people with self-reliance. People with low self-esteem and a reluctance to accept a challenge create a situation which allows others to control and make decisions for them.

Thirty-five-year-old Patty Brown, who must use a wheelchair because of an automobile accident at age sixteen, lived with her seventy-nine-year-old mother. Many times Patty's social worker and rehabilitation counselor urged her to move into a different living situation, and offered to compensate a person to help her learn how to cook and do the laundry. Each time, Patty refused the offer, giving the excuse that she felt unable to cope. Then one day, as they were eating lunch, her mother cried out. She clutched her chest and walked into the living room, but before reaching the sofa, she fell, dying of a heart attack.

Patty phoned her social worker and sobbed, "Mother is dead! Mother is dead! How am I going to get along by myself?" The social worker came to the house and decided to have the girl committed to a mental health facility, there was no other placement available on such short notice. In the hospital, the treatment staff observed that Patty was depressed and wanted assistance with her personal needs. They decided to place Patty in a convalescent hospital where she would receive proper care, and to appoint a guardian to oversee her financial and legal matters.

While her mother was still living, Patty experienced a life of comfort without considering the future. After her mother's death, Patty was unprepared to care for herself. She had created a situation where someone had to care for her. It is important for the handicapped to deal with their disabilities early and improve their condition to the greatest degree possible.

This chapter has discussed some of the reasons why it is of the highest priority for an individual with physical injuries to approve of those limitations and develop a positive attitude toward life. These case histories illustrate that the failure to make an adjustment can sometimes result in dire consequences. So, it is the purpose of this book to assist you in accepting the reality of your handicap as a means of helping you become a worthwhile individual despite your human condition.

Points to Remember

1. <u>Acceptance of your handicap is necessary</u>
<u>for good mental health:</u> Negative reactions such as anger, guilt, and depression can hamper peace of mind.

2. <u>Destructive feelings tend to interfere with a person's</u> <u>alertness:</u> Maladjustments to physical limitations can cause such interference.

3. <u>A disabled individual's well-being can affect physical</u> <u>health:</u> Negative reaction may impede bodily functioning.

4. <u>Acknowledging one's impairments and living with</u> <u>them positively promotes social acceptance.</u>

5. <u>Successful educational and vocation rehabilitation</u> <u>depend on how someone perceives his or her disabilities:</u> An individual must be willing and dedicated to improving the situation.

6. <u>The degree of people's physical independence and the</u> <u>ability to care for themselves is determined to a large extent by</u> <u>their motivation and appraisal of abilities:</u> A feeling of low personal value may bring about an individual's unnecessary dependence upon others.

Chapter 2
The Process of Acceptance

Previously, we discussed how Shelly, a high school cheerleader, who had been involved in an automobile accident, reacted after learning her spinal cord had been severed.

Once she had been active, running and jumping. Now, paralyzed from the neck down, she would spend the rest of her days either in a wheelchair or lying in bed with nurses attending to her every need around the clock.

Accepting handicaps is a challenge. For some, it is a life-long endeavor. Books have been written, including this one, about how to cope with such conditions. While these are helpful, the process of coping with our bodily limitations can be quite difficult. Even though many of us, including this author, know of ways to maintain good mental health, applying them takes continued effort.

Stages of Acceptance

In 1969, Dr. Elizabeth Kubler-Ross wrote the book: <u>ON DEATH AND DYING</u>. Death and a physical disability have something in common—a sense of loss. Death means you lose your life. An impairment means you lose your ability to perform as others do. With this in mind, consider these five stages of acceptance regarding your disability.

Denial: The first reaction that people who are disadvantaged may encounter is one of denial. They simply do not want to acknowledge that physical limitations exist. This was the case with Jeff, star quarterback of his high school football team.

During one of the Homecoming games, an opponent made a tackle, and Jeff fell to the ground. When he didn't get up, an ambulance was called. As the paramedics placed him on a stretcher, all four of his limbs appeared to be affected. He was moved to the emergency room, and the medical staff took X-rays.

A day later, his doctor came into the room, and said, "Jeff, your spinal cord was damaged. You are paralyzed and will be unable to use your legs and arms."
Jeff said, "Oh no, Doc, you must have looked at the X-rays wrong. I will be well in a few days."

Even with regular counseling by doctors and nurses, it was almost a month before Jeff accepted the fact that he would not have the full use of his arms and legs again.

Anger: Once a person realizes his or her injury is permanent, a sense of denial is replaced by one of anger. Often an individual is critical of the able-bodied because of envy. This was a problem with Jack, a quadriplegic, who went to camp at the suggestion of his counselor. It was thought that the experience might improve his outlook on life. However, Jack did not really want to go. He felt that most disadvantaged people were inferior and shouted to his mother, "I don't want to associate with those cripples!

"Now, now Jack," she replied, "Your attitude distresses me."

At camp Jack had a behavior problem. One morning while a counselor was trying to help him dress, he yelled, "Can't you do anything right? Your hurting me. I wish I could walk out of this hell hole."

Nothing anybody could do would satisfy Jack. This was not what others did, but Jack simply took his anger out on them, because of his own disability.

Bargaining: Bargaining occurs as the person attempts to postpone facing the fact that he or she has a disability. Such an individual is looking for a quick fix, or magic cure, or divine intervention in the hopes of a full recovery. Consider the following examples.

Ten-year-old Tony lay in the hospital recovering from an automobile accident. The doctors told his parents that he would be bedfast for the rest of his life. However, whenever his mother visited, Tony would remark, "Mommy, I know I will wake up well. A fairy told me."

This also takes place with those with a deep religous faith. For example, Barbara who was also paralyzed, went to the altar every Sunday at church. She really believed God would intervene, but was never healed. Thus she began to feel forgotten and started losing her faith.

Depression: Depression is an emotion many people face. Some cope with it successfully, but for others it is an on-going struggle.   In the remainder of this book, we will be dealing with ways to feel good about ourselves. Bear in mind, living with a disability requires patience and persistence. Depression can come and stay awhile. It's OK not to feel OK sometimes, as long as you are making an effort to accept your physical limitations.

Acceptance: The last stage in this process is acceptance. Each one of us must be able to "live with ourselves", or we will be miserable creatures and life will be robbed of its fullness and joy.

Allow Sufficient Time to Pass

As we have seen in the "Stages of Acceptance" it takes time to accept a disability. Here are four reasons why.

Physical Changes Occur: When you are involved in an accident or your condition becomes progressively worse, physical restoration may be required.   You might even need therapy for walking again, using an artificial limb, or maneuvering a wheelchair.   Rehabilitation may take days, weeks, and even months. For instance, a housewife who has a family and was paralyzed in a car accident, must learn housekeeping and child care skills from the position of a wheelchair.

Psychological Changes Are Occurring: No one who suffers from reduced bodily functioning can go through it without some psychological adjustment. After all, you have changed. There has been a loss. You will always have a picture of how you were before your injury or degeneration of health. Now you must look realistically at the body you have. You may have a desire for your condition to be reversed. You may mourn. You may cry. You may even want to die. These are all understandable emotions, but ones you must be willing to work on. The first step for a healthy outlook is the desire to distance yourself from any negative emotions you have had.

Don't Be Too Hard On Yourself: Don't become too self-critical because you cannot bounce back quickly with a positive attitude. Friends and relatives might try to cheer you by pointing out what other individuals have accomplished and what they have done with their lives. You still must come to terms with your injury. For example, it is agonizing to remember how it was to run, jump, and walk, while now knowing you will need to use a wheelchair the rest of your life, or face a daily battle with pain. In such situations, the tendency to display negative emotions is natural. Don't be depressed over being depressed. But there is a time to let go of your depression and to get on with your life.

<u>Give Yourself Permission:</u> Give yourself permission not to feel happy and joyful. People have the idea they must feel good all the time. This is a trap we can fall into by thinking that it is abnormal to be unhappy. Give yourself permission for mood swings.

Overcoming Excessive Negatives

In the previous section, we stated that it was all right to feel hurt and despondent about your condition. You are different than a majority of other people. Life will be more complicated for you. You might frequently need to cope with periods of despair.

This is the reality of the situation. However, the answer to feeling better does not stop with surrendering to the fact that you must go on living with a downcast attitude. You have probably heard that it is not the circumstances, but the way you react to the situation that determines the end result. Of course, this is easier said than done; however, in order to lead the most joyful life possible you should start your process of acceptance soon. You have been hurt, but you can bounce back. You have that ability. In the following pages, are ideas on how to live with yourself despite your physical limitations. These suggestions can make your emotional recovery easier.

Complete or Partial Acceptance

Is it possible to completely accept your impairments? This has been debated for sometime. Depending on what authority you listen to, the response could be different. One television personality interviewed a number of Miss America contestants who stated they all had found some unhappiness with their appearance. If these contestants have trouble with total acceptance, is it any wonder that someone disadvantaged would also have problems?

Perhaps you will never entirely accept your condition. In fact, this is a desire that may be unrealistic. Few people live on one big high all the time. The able-bodied experience emotional highs and lows. If this is true about those without physical ailments, don't expect perfection with yourself and remember that it is OK not to feel OK now and then.

You should strive to gain a partial acceptance of the situation. Make it a project to feel good about whatever you are experiencing, regardless of the circumstances. You may not be totally satisfied with the result, but at least you can have a reasonable amount of pleasure. Never forget that by being miserable, not only are you making yourself unhappy, but you are denying others the gifts of your talents and abilities which you could be using to help them.

Dependence Versus Independence

In chapter one, we mentioned the case of Patty Brown who used a wheelchair and had low self-esteem. Since she would not try to do anything for herself, when her mother died, the court appointed a guardian, and she was placed in a convalescent hospital. By not accepting some responsibility and continuing to wallow in self-pity, the only other option was for her to be cared for by the staff of an institution.

Dependence Means Surrendering: Dependence means surrendering control to others.

Personal Restrictions: For instance, if you were to live in a convalescent home under the care of a conservator, the facility would require many personal restrictions.

First, there might be rules on when to get up in the morning and also when to retire. Secondly, others plan your diet and how much food you will eat. Thirdly, patients may not be groomed properly. Some, in such residences, have gone without a bath for weeks.

IF YOU HAVE

HOPE

YOU CAN

COPE

Financial Restrictions: Those who relinquish control of their lives to others experience financial limitation. Often they are only given a small amount of money to spend for their own pleasures, and the rest of the income to which they are entitled, goes to a trustee and a convalescent facility, that usually charges inflated costs for their care.

Social Restrictions: There could be many social restrictions connected with being dependent on other people. For instance, a handicapped individual may not be able to make decisions without consulting someone else first about the plans.

Mental Restrictions: Often those in the care of others only hear one side of a story which may or may not be true. For example, state investigators visit convalescent hospitals periodically to investigate the quality of care. At one of these institutions, the staff brought the patients together. One staff member remarked, "You better be careful what you say during the visit, or you might lose your home."

Legal Restrictions: When you are receiving aid from caretakers and on conservatorship, you are deemed not legally responsible. For instance, you cannot enter into contracts alone. You cannot get married, since this act is a contract, without having the permission of another.

Independence Means Control.

Living with physical problems does present a challenge. Sometimes you may feel like giving up and being cared for by someone else. On the surface this may look appealing, but when you consider the restraints that may be demanded, does not independence seem like a more positive alternative?

Points To Remember

1. There are five stages of acceptance: These include: denial, anger, bargaining, depression, and acceptance.

2. Allow sufficient time to pass: Physical changes occur. Psychological problems come about. Don't be too frustrated. Give yourself permission to experience frustration or sadness.

3. Overcome excessive negativism: The longer you dwell on negative thoughts, the tougher it is to think positive.

4. Some people may accept their limitations to a greater degree than others: It is difficult to be happy with yourself continuously. You may experience mood swings

5. Dependence versus independence: Dependence means surrender of control to others. Independence involves freedom to make personal choices.

6. You must decide to accept your disability.

Chapter 3

There Are No Easy Answers

Diane McGinty, born with cerebral palsy, lay in the hospital with her left foot tightly bandaged with gauze. Only the day before, she had pushed the joy stick of her electric wheelchair with her chin and intentionally propelled herself into a sliding glass door, hoping to cut herself severely so that she would bleed to death.

Mrs. Ross, an ill-tempered social worker walked into Diane's room, leaned over the bed and with a harsh voice, asked, "Why did you try suicide?"

Responding in low, garbled tones, Diane mumbled, "I wanted to die."

Mrs. Rose quickly added, "I can't understand what you are saying! Here's your word board."

Holding a stick tightly between her lips, Diane pointed to each of the letters which formed words in a sentence, "I feel worthless. I am useless."

In a non-compassionate manner, Mrs. Rose exclaimed, "Stop the pity trip! Just cheer up!" With these words, she turned and stalked out of the room.

Easy answers. Simple solutions. Hollow promises. These are some of the approaches used by professionals who were employed to serve the disabled.

In Diane's case, she had studied six years to earn a degree in psychology. Soon after obtaining the B.A. degree, her parents were accidentally killed. Since she could not care for herself, the young woman was placed in a community care facility with mentally retarded individuals, where nurses dressed, bathed, and fed everyone. Diane had thought her education would lead to a job. She longed for public contact; she wanted to feel worthwhile. Instead, she just sat in a nursing facility, watching Soap Operas and game shows on television day after day, grieving in depression.

Many others along with Diane, who have brilliant minds but with severe handicaps, also have desires and aspirations like anyone else. They may have difficult questions; the questions may seem to defy solutions, but nevertheless are justified. Remember though, there are often no easy answers to some of those queries. We all want to be happy with our life circumstance. So, when considering such issues as are discussed in this chapter, it is wise to do that in a realistic and positive manner.

Why Me?

Asking yourself this question indicates that you have not yet accepted your impairments. But do not misinterpret this statement as a condemnation. Realizing you are different is difficult; it makes most of us uncomfortable.

Four years ago, John Williams, born with cerebral palsy, was still able to walk. Then one morning, as he waited outside the bank for the doors to open his legs and hips began to hurt. Intense pain ran up and down both legs, as he stood on one then the other. Soon his condition worsened to the point he had to be hospitalized, and it was determined that he had three slipped discs in the lower back which could not be sufficiently treated. As a result, he would be confined to a wheelchair for life. Even though considerable time has passed, when John wakens in the morning and sees his wheelchair, since he remembers what it was like to have the freedom of mobility and is sad.

This is not an unusual reaction. It is normal to wish you were able-bodied. However, to agonize because you can no longer accomplish certain things, is unhealthy and may bring about mental distress. Some people habitually live in the past, thinking if they had not done "this or that," they would not have had injuries. There is no point living with regrets; the past is gone forever, the future is yet to be. A very special friend said to me, "Look at what you have left, not what you have lost."

Will Everything Be Fine?

Frequently, those working with the limited, attempt to "paint a rosy picture" by saying, "Everything will be fine." This is over-simplification. The more severe your condition, the more discomforts you will have. There will be both physical and psychological adjustments. Life-style changes may be needed. There could be pain, difficult interpersonal relationships and discrimination. Certainly, there will be circumstances requiring much time and effort to resolve.

There might not be any simple results at hand for the situations confronting some, but be positive. Bill Tibia, a mental health counselor, once said, "There is always an answer. We may not know what it is, when needed but there is an answer."

Is Life Worth Living?

A few years ago, a national news story dealt with Elizabeth Bovia, a cerebral-palsied, young woman who had a Master of Arts Degree, and who was extremely depressed. At the time Elizabeth was hospitalized, and refused to eat. The medical staff fed her through a tube to keep her alive. Elizabeth had no use of her arms or legs, and was totally dependent on others for personal care. She had decided that she no longer wanted to live and went to court to seek the right to die. In accordance with the law, the judge denied her request.

Is life worth living for someone so incapacitated? Is suicide an option to consider? Let's attempt to take a logical look at this question. We must assume that there will be readers of this book who believe in God and those that do not. Certainly, belief in a higher power has not been proven conclusively. Since many of us are undecided, why not be safe and suppose He does exist. The ten commandments tell us, "Thou Salt Not Kill." In his book, God's Way To A God Life.

Dr. Robert Schuller, a minister of renown, states, "Suicide is the murder of self. Perhaps the church has been too reticent on this issue. We do not want to offend others, so we courteously avoid calling attention to what the Bible says on this subject: "No murderer....shall enter into the kingdom of heaven." This fear of the consequences has probably stopped many people from killing themselves."

Aside from the religious aspect, one must always consider that medical discoveries are being brought about at an accelerating pace, and it is unbelievable what the future could bring regarding cures of various illnesses and the alleviation of others.

To What Extent Can I Be Rehabilitated?

This depends on your impairments. Listen carefully to your doctors, nurses, and therapists. Be certain you heare what they say, not what you want to hear.

Depending on the circumstance, you might want to have a second opinion or a third. This is not skepticism. It is intelligence. After all, you want to be sure you are doing all you can for yourself. In the case of recommended surgery, you should be convinced that it is really needed, or in all likelihood will be beneficial.

Work with your therapists. Follow their instructions as carefully as you can. Give no heed to outsiders who may indicate you are not trying. Most people have no idea about the struggle you are having.

Finally, face reality and acknowledge your physical limitations. As stated in the first chapter, for the sake of your own mental health, you must emotionally adjust to your condition.

If you were told that you will probably never walk again, there would be no advantage in spending time wishing you might awaken one morning and discover yourself walking.

Chuck Tolbert, a quadriplegic, told the story of how he had his attendant place him in the middle of the floor, stand him upright, and then no longer hold him. Chuck took one step and fell. Later he realized how foolish he had been, and that he must accept his situation.

How Can I Cope With My Disability

Is it possible for handicapped persons to fully accept themselves? At times it seems so challenging. But this is an aim that can be achieved depending on the individual and the extent of his or her involvement.

Dr. Robert Merkle, executive director of Christian Counseling Services, Inc., made the following statement some years ago: "Positive thinking is the world's biggest con job. For that matter, negative thinking is also a con job."

Now, what did Dr. Merkle really mean? He could have meant that not one of us, no matter how brilliant, is capable of predicting the future with any accuracy. Even the most highly educated professor cannot foresee the accomplishments of a truly dedicated person with multiple injuries.

Here are some guidelines that have helped me cope when I felt really overwhelmed. First, one should recognize your disabilities are real. In my case, I must use a wheelchair. Secondly, while acknowledging that bodily conditions exist, do not minimize your ability to overcome or compensate for them. Finally, don't establish goals too low for yourself. Instead, go forward, always striving to obtain your maximum. Often you can accomplish more than you think.

What About My Educational Future

Michael James, sixteen, was a straight A student in high school and had plans to attend college and major in law. One afternoon on the way home from school, he was involved in an automobile accident which paralyzed him from the neck down. He wondered if he still could attend college, or was his dream of continuing his education impractical now.

Today, opportunities are increasing for those who are physically limited; many of the large colleges and universities have Enabling Programs to assist students. They offer a number of services. Blind students are often supplied with readers. Those who are deaf can frequently be assigned a Sign Language Interpreter. For anyone having difficulty writing, tests can be given orally. In other words, higher educational institutions are providing more accomodations for this type of student.

Can I Find A Suitable Vocation?

In the area of employment there is good and bad news. Today, more job opportunities exist for the physically disabled. One example is that the California State Personnel Board has developed the Limited Examination and Employment Program to assist individuals in obtaining Civil Service positions in the California State Government. LEAP, as the program is referred to, consists of a series of job classifications especially for those who are disadvantaged.

However, for the group of individuals having speech difficulty, finding a placement will often require much patience. The problem can be compounded if the applicant has mobility, hand, or arm limitations.

As an illustration, many people with cerebral palsy earn college degrees and yet are unable to obtain a job. For years, this has been a challenge to vocational rehabilitation professionals. A solution to consider is a Home Operated Business. There are many different types of services. Some ideas are home typing, a telephone reminding service, sign making, and compiling a Baby Sitting Registry for those who might be interested. More information can be obtained by contacting: Accent On Information, P.O. Box 700, Bloomington, Illinois 61701.

Is Independent Living Possible?

If you have a strong determination, and were born with a disability or acquired one later in life, you can live independently. To begin with, we must understand what is meant by independent living. In my earlier book The Disabled Homemaker, I defined independent living by quoting the explanations of Joel Bryant, who uses a wheel chair and is director of Disabled Student's Programs at the University of California, Davis, California.

Joel stated his ideathis way: "For me it really means autonomous living; someone having the ability to direct his or her life even though the person cannot perform all the necessary tasks. This involves accepting responsibility and being sufficiently competent to plan your life."

Although the individual may require additional help, he or she can live independently, if the person can hire and fire attendants appropriately. Consequently, arranging for reliable attendant care may be an important factor to consider when determining the ability to live in your own home or apartment.

Points To Remember

1. <u>Asking "Why me?", is a waste of time and mental energy</u> Don't live with regrets.

2. <u>Your situation may be difficult:</u> Your problems may seem unsolvable. You may not know the solution, but keep searching. There are answers.

3. <u>Find life worth living:</u> Suicide is a risk. Death could be worse than the pain of your condition.

4. <u>Rehabilitate yourself to the fullest extent possible then try to accept the areas that cannot be changed:</u> Have hope.

5. <u>You can psychologically adjust:</u> Remain optimistic.

6. <u>Continue your learning:</u> Many educational institutions offer programs for students who are limited. More opportunities are becoming available. Don't be a quitter.

Chapter 4
Dealing With The Feelings

Having a disability is not only a physically but also emotionally disturbing experience. There is an old expression, "You don't know what it is like until you walk in the other person's shoes."

Many people who attempt to counsel those with severe limitations do not always understand the individual's true feelings. They attempt to apply "Band-Aid" solutions to very complex situations. Trite phrases such as: "There, there now, everything will be all right," are often given in haste. For example, Barbara attends a church, and each Sunday, she lies in her reclining wheelchair. When she tries to speak, her words are garbled. During the week, she lives in a convalescent hospital where the staff is often verbally abusive. Her well-intentioned friends simply say words such as, "It's OK. Hope. Just smile." Wouldn't it be wonderful if resolving situations would be that easy? Unfortunately, most times they are not.

General Considerations

Before discussing negative emotions, here is some general information that can apply to psychological problems handicapped people may face.

Negative Emotions Are Natural: This may sound contrary to all good counseling suggestions, but let's be practical. Consider the following illustration. Seventeen-year-old Betty was a high school cheerleader, an 'A' student, and planning to become a doctor. She was also an equestrian who had won many ribbons and trophies in competition. One day while Betty was preparing for a show, her horse heard a shrill noise and bucked. The girl was thrown to the ground and taken to the hospital. After taking X-rays, it was determined she would never walk again. It took Betty many months to adjust emotionally to her impairments. She was depressed and unhappy.

If someone experiences a negative emotional reaction, what does that mean? For instance, when a person is depressed, are the words, "cheer up" apt to cause the individual to do so immediately? Usually not. Emotions are indicators that something is physically or mentally wrong. A counselor trained in working with people with impairments should try to uncover the cause of the problem. Superficial answers to complex problems won't help. They may only create a greater difficulty. The reasons for the situations should be addressed, not merely the negative feelings themselves.

Other People's Perceptions: Why not be honest with one another? How do people view someone with a disability? Here is a list of adjectives: helpless, dependent, poor cripple, pitiful. This list could be endless. The point is many persons have a negative opinion of someone limited. While there are many disadvantaged employed, there also are a greater number of individuals who do not obtain jobs, even though they are qualified. A quadriplegic with a law degree had much trouble finding a firm to hire him simply because he used a wheelchair.

Professionals and non-professionals alike can have this view. Michael Jones, who had a speech impediment and other disabilities, sat in a Sunday School class. Mr. Cole, a Marriage, Family and Child counselor, told the group how he wrote freelance articles. After the session, Michael approached him and in a mumbling tone of voice began telling him that he was a writer too, and wanted to discuss the business with him. Mr. Cole, although polite, felt uncomfortable and thought, "He probably can't write a sentence much less a book." A few weeks later, Michael wrote Mr. Cole a letter, asking some questions about writing. The Sunday School teacher was ashamed that he had initially formed such a wrong impression of the young man.

Our Self Perceptions: Both the Russian psychologist Pavalov and B.F. Skinner, believed in the theory of conditioning. Their idea is that our reactions reflect our experiences. Is it any wonder that many handicapped people have emotional problems, since able-bodied people relate to them often in a condescending way. Be careful when listening to the negative counsel of others. They may be under-estimating your abilities. Often handicapped people can do more than first seems possible.

Aside from the negative impact others have on those with impediments, the injured will consider their limitations and wonder if the struggle to improve is worth the effort. They may look inward at what they cannot do instead of focusing on personal abilities and the future that is still before them.

TOUGH TIMES

WILL NOT LAST

TOUGH PEOPLE DO

You can only change yourself: Frequently, diabled people become bitter and believe they are experiencing discrimination. Of course, not everyone relates to the less able with respect and equality. However, one should remember this cardinal rule: "You can only change yourself." When we experience a negative situation, someone once said, "It is not the circumstance that is troubling, but your reaction to it." Therefore, it is helpful to be cognizant of your response and make alterations in beneficial ways.

The Downward Slide: The problem of refusing to deal with negative emotions is that you allow them to engulf your life. These conditions can become unpleasant. You will experience a downward slide from being happy to living in the pits of despair. In so doing, you not only endure psychological problems, but physical ones as well. Continual stress can cause ulcers, or intense rage could bring on a heart attack, resulting in death.

Specific Emotions

Victimization
Another word for victimization is self-pity. To begin with, let's review two of the conditions discussed earlier in this chapter how others perceive those with limitations, and how we view ourselves. Remember those negative descriptive adjectives—hopeless, dependent, poor cripple, helpless? If a person is perceived as anyu of these, it is only natural they will feel like

victims. Consequently, it follows that the individual pities his-selves. If parents of a handicapped son or daughter react to him or her in a disparaging way and underestimate the child's abilities, the person will most likely develop the same attitude about him or herself. This is only logical.

But how can you rise above your feelings of hopelessness? Here are five ways:

1. Determine Victimization Is Wrong: Even though you may have a strong tendency to want sympathy, make the desision that it is wrong. This can be the beginning of a change in attitude. You can feel like a victim if you choose, but this will not help improve your situation. Connie Black, a Senior Mental Health worker, reminds her clients that times may be tough, but you must be strong enough to take the guff. Everyone should learn to be strong in adversity. It serves no useful purpose to whine and become bitter. So show courage.

2. Establish Who You Are: Do you think of yourself as a loser or winner in life? Do you control your circumstances, or do they control you? To illustrate these points, here are two examples:

Bob a quadriplegic, who was injured in a football accident, seldom gets out of bed. He spends his time drinking beer and watching television. He has no motivation to become self-supporting.

On the other hand, Edward V. Roberts, also a quadriplegic who uses a respirator as a result of polio, founded the Center for Independent Living in Berkeley, California, and later was appointed California State Director of the Department of Rehabilitation.

The idea is that often a disabled person can do more than either themselves or others think they can. Your mental attitude determines if you will become a victim or victor.

3. Decide To Be A Conqueror: Deciding you will try to do something is really a choice. On the subject of decision making, there are only two alternatives: either "you will" or "you won't." Even not making a choice is a determination to do nothing. If you attempt something, in the process, you build self-esteem, dignity and hope. If you try to eliminate all chance of achievement you miss the joy that comes with making an effort. What if you are defeated? You can always try again. This will be dealt with further in chapter five.

4. Reject Negative Input: Mary Crane had polio when she was young and used underarm crutches, but this 'A' student had a goal of becoming a doctor. Her professors in Medical School discouraged her. Today, despite her limitations she is performing surgery in one of this nation's hospitals.

A detrimental type of rehabilitation professional is one who tells you what you can't do rather than what you can do. While they are regarded as experts, some of them only confuse and do not solve the problems. So don't listen to such negative input. If you feel reasonably certain that you can fulfill a desire, go forward and try.

6. Isolate Yourself From Defeatisim: Joe Fry, an eighteen-year-old honor student, planned to attend college and become an accountant. One day, while the senior was driving home from high school, he lost control of his car and veered into an abutment, resulting in paralysis. After being released from the hospital, he soon realized that his parents related to him differently.

One night Joe's drunken mother and father began arguing with him. "We were so proud of you," his mother said. "Now look at you; you're a hopeless cripple." Joe replied, "I still want to go to college. I still think I can make a good accountant." "Joe", his father laughed, "you will never get through school, much less fill a position. Get that idea out of your stupid head. Here, I will help you," and slapped him across the back, and added, "You are now a disgrace to the human race."

The following Monday morning, Joe told his counselor about the incident and expressed a desire to move out of the home. A social worker helped make the arrangements, and Joe never again had any contact with his uncaring parents. Their company was damaging to his well-being.

Sometimes for your own mental health, you must cut off those who have negative opinions of you. In some cases, isolating yourself from such individuals may be the best alternative.

Rejection

We have already mentioned how people often reject and treat the disabled unfairly. This is a fact, so one must learn to adjust. Attitudes are difficult to change.

Abusive Behavior Cannot Be Helped: You cannot control what other people do to you. For instance, Mike Ronald, was born with cerebral palsy, had only a slight speech impairment, and was brilliant. He earned his undergraduate degree in a small midwestern town, and then moved to California. After his first semester, when in a staff conference, Wanda Williams, a professor, told him in an abrupt tone of voice, "There is no use for you continuing in this program. Your disability prevents you from counseling. You are unemployable. This department will not assist you in finding placement. You would be wasting our time." This type of rejection can be devastating if you let it. You have encountered another person who has not yet learned to be tactful.

Abusive Behavior Can Hurt: No one likes rejection. There are two ways that people often react to this. They are either "blowing up" or "claming up." When you clam up, you may experience victimization. When you blow up you lash out in anger. Neither way is emotionally beneficial for you. There are other alternatives.

Abusive Behavior Can Be Healed: and you can achieve peace and happiness in the process. First, abusive behaivior can be healed, analyze how you feel, and how emotionally destructive the other person's behavior or remarks seemed. Secondly, forgive the individual. Don't continually rehash the thing over in your mind. The last chapter of this book will cover this topic in-depth. Thirdly, when you cannot escape abuse, learn to live with it.

Anger

Does anger really pay? To answer this question, why not examine how this emotion affects you personally. There are two ways: physically and psychologically. Anger can bring about adverse conditions such as high-blood pressure, ulcers and indigestion. In some instances, headaches may occur. The disabled should not compound their limitations with such health problems. There can also be disturbed mental functioning. People in this state of mind tend to think unclearly and make irrational judgments. Almost daily, someone appears in our nation's courts accused of horrible crimes, and makes a plea of insanity. Sometimes they were intensely angry when the offense was committed.

Not only will anger have a devastating effect on one's well-being, it can also have an influence with personal friendships. Few of us enjoy communicating with someone who is angry. It is acceptable to have a disagreement with another and to express it in a civilized way. Debate is healthy. However, it is a different matter to physically and emotionally abuse those who oppose you. After all, everyone is entitled to an opinion.

Is anger ever justified? Of course. There are intolerable conditions that should be rectified and in those situations change must take place. The problem then becomes: how to alter the circumstances with the least amount of mental distress. Here are four suggestions to minimize anger and have healthy relationships with others.

1. Control Your Temper: Whatever the problem may be and however much abuse you are taking, try to remain in charge of your emotions. Be cautious when speaking, as you may have regrets later. Remember, there are times when the length of your conversation or the quality of evidence does not always convince everyone. In these confrontations, it is really a waste of time to try changing the mind of another who becomes hostile.

2. Calculate Your Response: Be calm and think about the situation. You may be faced with correcting a wrong.

Would you really want to do it quickly? Instead of acting inappropriately, pause and examine with care some means of coping with the matter to maintain good results and minimize stress.

Distrust Negative Impressions: When someone differs with you, refrain from labeling them. Be sure that you give the individual a fair hearing and listen closely while he or she speaks. Often we believe we understand what motivates a person and we really do not. When this is found to be true, our misjudgment has been erroneous and will only serve to further strain a relationship.

How important is the issue? Rather than becoming angry, ask yourself: "How important is the issue?" Quite frequently people will become disturbed over minor things that really do not make a significant difference. For instance, two men argued about whether a car that passed them on the street was green or blue. One was irate when he wasn't successful in making his point. His acquaintance became aware that it was trivial to pursue that discussion further and promptly changed the subject.

Anger hampers clear thinking while staying calm allows adequate time to proceed with problem solving.

A WISE MAN

KEEPS HIS ANGER

UNDER CONTROL

Hostility

Hostility is anger acted out. You may be distraught and want to punch someone in the nose. You become hostile when you act on that thought. Some psychologists recommend that people vent their emotions to keep from becoming depressed, while Christians indicate that hostility is a violation of the love principle. Jesus Christ said "Love your neighbor as yourself." But why not choose learning to control your anger, so it will not become hostility? Here are two good reasons:

1. Physical Well-Being: When you become hostile, your physical appearance changes. For example, a man with gait problems, when taunted may become more clumsy because he is angry.
2. Bodily Danger: A disabled person who attempts to use violence against an able-bodied person often puts himself in physical danger. There is a good reason for this. Often a person without limitations is stronger and has more control than one with limitations. Always consider that often a non-disabled person has the advantage over someone with impairments.

Envy

Fifteen-year-old Tommy, sitting in a wheelchair, paralyzed as a result of a plane crash, watched his friends play baseball. Only two years before, he had been standing at first base, hitting strikes and making home runs.

Being envious of his friends, Tommy turned to one of the players and said "Why did it happen to me—not the other guy?" It is quite understandable why this youth was agitated, but such feelings have negative consequences.

Envy Focuses On What Is Lost: Some disabilities cannot be corrected; a person who envies someone able-bodied, wishes for something that cannot be. The constant and prolonged desire for what is not possible, only complicates the acceptance of one's future likelihood for progress.

Envy Produces Anger: Jealousy develops feelings of anger towards our fellow man. Previously, I had explained the implications of anger on daily living. It can impair interpersonal relationships; it also demonstrates you have not adjusted to your limitations.

Envy Hampers Forward Thinking: If you are jealous and resentful of others, if you spend your time comparing their life circumstance to yours, your creative abilities may be blocked. Why not concentrate on the aptitudes you now possess, rather than wasting time on what might have been.

Fear And Worry

In her senior year of college, Betty Morgan lost her balance and fall. During the Christmas season, while shopping, she collapsed and was taken to the hospital where her doctor performed an MRI Scan. When the results were in, the physician told her she had Multiple Sclerosis. This could mean she would eventually be confined to a wheelchair or bed with reduced bodily functions. Death could occur within ten to twenty years. Betty becameworried and fearful because her body was wasting away.

This woman's reaction is comprehensible, but the emotion of fear can cripple individuals psychologically so they cannot function normally.

The Relationship Of Stress: What causes the stress of fear? It is sometimes unpredictable. We all want to direct our future. When we lose the power over our personal lives, we tend to panic. In Betty's case, she no longer could depend on good health and was unable to do much to deter her failing physical condition.

Worry And Uncertainty: According to Dr. Robert Merkle, Executive Director of the Christian Counseling Services, Inc., "Worry is something one does when he or she may not know what would be the best course of action to take."

Falsehoods And Fear: Following is a falsehood that encourages fear. People have the mistaken idea that all human conditions are manageable. Certainly this is not true.

Someone with AIDS faces death in the future, since there is no medical cure for the ailment at this time. Obviously, an AIDS patient cannot manage the progression of the affliction.

The Key Of Surrender: In World War II, millions of Jews were imprisoned in German concentration camps. Daily, they lived with the fear of death. Many innocent victims starved, were executed, and tortured. Corri Tambone was one of the prisoners. Hourly, she watched her fellow cell mates die. Certainly, this was a horrifying situation. There was nothing she could do to change her environment. She was helpless. After Corri realized this, she decided to try having faith and trust that better things would come. Along with this decision came peace— a peace and well-being that could cope with whatever her situation.

In such cases, one should remember we do have control over some things in our lives, but in some circumstances we are powerless and helpless. As earlier indicated, AIDS patients face death. Death could be classified as the Final Fear, or, is it merely a transition into another state of existence. Some say, this is possible or even probable. The key is then surrender to fate of faith in God. This is the choice of every reader of this book. But surrendering to something beyond yourself is the key to overcoming fear and experiencing peace of mind. Even though you can't fit all the pieces of your life in place, as you might choose, have faith things will work out for the best. In so doing, you allow peace to replace fear.

Anxiety

What causes anxiety? Why do people worry about choices in their lives?

Alternatives: Such confusion arises because the disabled sometimes face many alternatives. What doctor to choose? Should I remain on SSI, or seek employment? Should I have elective surgery? Such questions are difficult because if the decision should later prove to have not been in one's best interest, it can be emotionally disturbing.

Mistaken Belief: How does this happen? It is the mistaken belief that the correct action must always be taken to get the best results. What is the proper procedure? Have you ever heard, "The best laid plans sometimes go away?" For example, a few years ago the space shuttle, Challenger, was launched. At that time, shuttle launchings had almost become routine. Most people paid little attention to these events. However, on the day this shuttle was launched, a few minutes after lift-off, a red ball of flame appeared in the air. The craft was on fire. A blast killed the crew while the nation mourned in shock and disbelief.

Mistaken Desire: There is another erroneous thought that can lead to anxiety. Individuals have the notion that they must choose the right plan to chart their future. Such a person can be immobilized and have difficulty making a decision. How foolish! Do we expect a 100% guarantee in all matters? Sorry, that is unrealistic.

A Healthy Perspective: What we have been saying thus

far is that all events cannot be managed successfully, and it is not completely in our control for things to develop as expected. So then, how should we reduce anxiety? First, welcome opportunities available to you. NOTE the word <u>available</u>. Despite the best efforts, and even though you may think you have all the information at hand, there are unforeseen factors of which you are unaware. Then it is your task to pursue the options based on what is at hand, avoiding an attempt to predict the future. It is advantageous then to use the findings you have, and not be unduly concerned about anything that may arise.

Guilt

Tom Murry asked Diane Williams to marry him three times. She always refused and moved out of the city. Tom felt rejected and frequently thought of suicide. One day he walked into the middle of the street, was hit by a car but not killed. Instead, he was paralyzed in his lower extremities. After pondering for months over what had happened, he felt guilty about his previous action. In such situations, guilt serves no purpose. How do you deal with it? Here are three helpful, although not easy steps:

1. Agree That What You Did Was Wrong: in a constructive way, examine yourself and conclude that the experience was a mistake. In the case of suicide, it is legally, morally, and biblically unacceptable. Take it seriously. Don't make an excuse, or shift the blame. Shoulder your responsibility. You made an error.

2. Vow The Incident Will Never Happen Again: Promise yourself that you will never repeat the wrongful action.

The temptation may come, but you need not yield to it. You have great power—the power of self control. That is always an option.

3. Forgive Yourself: Acknowledge the fact, that you are not perfect. The late psychiatrist Dr. Theodore Reik, said "One can feel sorry about something without feeling guilty. A clear understanding of our misdeeds is emotionally healthier than hopeless misery afterwards."

Alienation

Often times, disabled people have difficulty relating to the able-bodied, as the following illustrates regarding Janet and Diane. "Janet, are you going to the dance tonight? Diane asked. "Who me? Of course not, Diane," Janet answered.

Janet had just returned to school after an automobile accident, which left her confined to a wheelchair. She thought she might be uncomfortable in a social environment.

"Now, Janet. Your are no different than before your injury," Diane said. "You are going to the dance! I will pick you up at 8:00. I don't want to hear any back talk from you."

If you have problems relating to the able-bodied, here are three guidelines that may help you.

1. We All Have Equal Rights: As we stated earlier, some who are handicapped feel like victims of discrimination. Even though others may not think you can do much, you must remember that just because you have a physical limitation, is no indication you haven't much potential. Refrain from thinking of yourself as inferior. Never forget it isn't the opinion of others that matters, it is how you evaluate yourself. So when you interact with someone who is without injury, remember that you have as much value and worth as the next person. You may have assets the other person does not have.

2. Mix And Mingle: Often it is difficult for an impaired person to associate with a non-impaired person. As an illustration; after a long hospitalization, Marie, was released. Having once been ambulatory, she now had to use a wheelchair, and could not wear shoes due to their weight which caused spinal pain. Consequently, the first time she went to church in a wheelchair without shoes, she felt very self-conscious. This is a normal reaction, but you must force yourself to socialize. You will find that as you mix and mingle, the feeling of alienation will slowly disappear.

3. Allow Others To Know You: Able-bodied people have many misconceptions about the physically limited. For one example, a person who has a speech problem may not be considered intelligent. We will discuss stereo types in chapter nine. Therefore, it is important that people experience our abilities instead of focusing on impairments. We have gifts and talents despite our impairments.

Depression

Earlier in this chapter, we explained the "Downward Slide." As mentioned before, if negative emotions are not corrected, they can take you from happiness to hopelessness. This is particularly true of depression. Suppose that there are eight stages of depression you can pass through from the beginning to the end of the slide. On your progress towards the end, you gradually move from joy to the depths of despair. When considering these stages, we will apply them to one individual and her emotional struggles.

Joyce, a sixteen-year-old cheerleader at Mortonville High School, went on a camp out with her boyfriend, John. They prepared to go swimming, and Joyce decided to dive from a rock into the edge of the lake below. Moments after hitting the water, her body floated to the top. John sensed there was something wrong and called out, "Are you all right?" There came no answer.

A man in a car called out, to John "Can I help?" John answered in a concerned voice, "My girlfriend is in trouble. Wait here. If I wave my hand, please call an ambulance."

Speedily, John swam out to Joyce. She was unconscious, and he waved for help and soon she was transported to the hospital with a serious, crippling injury.

The stages in relation to Joyce's injury and the events leading to her depression now follow.

Stage One – Impatience: When sick or injured, you are naturally impatient to know what has happened to your body. The problem arises when you suspect something is seriously wrong. In Joyce's case, after she regained consciousness, she could not move her legs or arms.

Stage Two – Anger: When in trauma and impatient, negative thoughts arise and anger can result.

One morning, Dr. Roberts walked into Joyce's room. "Hi Doc," said Joyce. "When do I start walking and feeding myself? When do I go home?" Grim-faced, Dr. Roberts said, "Joyce, you've got some long days of rehabilitation ahead. Your spinal cord was damaged at the C5 level. In other words you broke your neck. This means you can never expect to walk again. How much you will be able to use your arms is still unknown." Joyce cried out, "You can't be right. I will walk again." Dr. Roberts replied, "Sorry, I wish I could tell you otherwise, but we must face the medical reality."

After Dr. Roberts left the room, Joyce became angry. She was furious with herself for having dived in waters that were unknown to her. She had been warned that one cannot always know what is at the bottom of such places. She also seethed inside that a sign had not been posted to warn swimmers of such potential danger. It is important to deal constructively concerning the anger within yourself and the hostility toward others at this time.

Stage Three – Disappointment: When the moment comes that you know you must accept your disability, a struggle to cope with the reality begins. It is then time to prepare yourself with the battle of remaining positive. In Joyce's situation, this was not easy for her. She had once been a cheerleader, active and athletic ; it was difficult for her to realize that she would not be the same. There were times of crying and periods when she tried to acquire courage for the future. Joyce read some books: Joni and A Further Step by Joni Eareckson Tada who is a quadriplegic and Director of a religious nonprofit organization serving physically challenged people.

Stage Four – Discouragement: It is easy to become discouraged when you are physically limited. Not only do you fight the emotions from within; but you must also battle problems others may unintentionally create. For example, one day John came into Joyce's room and said, "Joyce, our engagement is off." "Why?" she questioned, "I thought you loved me." John said, "I did, but that was before..." "Before what?", Joyce exclaimed. "You know. The accident. I just can't handle it. You in a wheelchair; it just won't work out. I'm sorry Joyce. Good-bye". John then left the room.

Stage Five – Disillusionment: At this point, the individual experiences a feeling of being let down. With Joyce, when her boyfriend left, she felt deserted and wondered if she was still a person of value now that she was physically injured. Joyce began to doubt her self-worth.

WHEN IN THE

PIT OF DESPAIR

HANG IN

THERE!

Stage Six – Victimization: We dealt with victimization previously in this chapter, but now I want to tie it into the "Downward Slide" to depression. To feel victimized is probably one of the most contributing factors to depression. In this case, Joyce thought of herself as a victim and felt self-pity because of her physical limitations and rejection by her boy friend. After John broke off their relationship, Joyce wanted to die rather than live with her crippled body.

Stage Seven – Death: At least 50,000 to 70,000 people attempt suicide every year in the United States. Only a small percentage of those who try, actually succeed, but the guilt of having tried can create even more problems.

On going depression can damage one's physical and mental health. It is important to take action to prevent this. The process of restoration needs to begin to prevent a downward slide.

Withdrawal And Isolation

As stated earlier, Joni Eareckson Tade, a quadriplegic, has established a national ministry that touches the lives of thousands. Yet, there are many handicapped people who isolate themselves, spending their time at home, wasting life away.

What is the difference between Joni and the others? It is a simple decision to fight the tough battles. That isn't easy. The struggle to avoid becoming a "closet cripple" is hard. As we move toward the year 2000, disabled people are among those whom society discriminate against the most. We have the choice to succumb or overcome. Time must be given to achieve recognition, but there is no good reason for isolating yourself or be withdrawn. Even those who are homebound can invite friends to visit them. Why not decide to be a doer, not a closet cripple for the welfare of yourself and others. You will surely reap rewards from your service as you help those in need.

Choosing A Counselor For You

Selecting a counselor to help you with your personal problems is often difficult but urgent. Some psychologists and mental health workers can make one so confused, the problems actually intensify. You will want to make sure the counseling is really beneficial. Here are some suggestions to assist making that determination:

1. Are you and your counselor compatible? Perhaps on your first meeting, you do not feel comfortable. There seems to be an atmosphere of impatience and the use of words you do not understand. The individual could be relating to you in a disparaging manner. He or she might be using offensive language that is distasteful to you. This is probably rare, but it does happen. If you really dislike your advisor, or feel uncombortable the time spent may not be of benefit. You must find someone you thrust and believe cares about you.

2. Do you value conflict? What are your values? Do you derive satisfaction from just recreation or from achievement? For instance; if the therapist is a pleasure-seeking Freudian type, he or she might belittle your desire for accomplishment.

The person could be an atheist and refuse any discussion of Christianity. (Note: you may be told by some agencies this is against the rules). Whatever the basic difference in thought, there could be a barrier to you receiving the help you need.

3. Is Your Counselor Too Impersonal?: If he or she seems distant or aloof, you may not be receiving the emotional warmth needed to promote personal growth. A therapist may try to mask his or her own inadequacies by keeping some emotional detachment, causing you to wonder if the person really cares.

4. When You Question The Advice Given: While it is wonderful to work with a charming counselor, there is one caution to bear in mind. Some people regard themselves as "all knowing gurus". When such a condition develops, it can rob one of objectivity by accepting the counselors point of view. This is a disadvantage because it prevents you from thinking for yourself.

5. Does Your Counselor Have "Hang-ups"?: If the counselor continues wanting to talk about issues that have little value to you, but seems important to the advisor, this may indicate that he or she is more concerned about meeting the needs of their ego rather than helping you.

6. Should Your Counselor Want To Control You:
Some professionals may want to control your behavior. Their interests may go far beyond psychological guidance. It is a well-known fact that some therapists have sexually abused their clients. There are instances where some have threatened the clients not to break away from the relationship because his or her emotional health could deteriorate. If such tactics are used, one should beware and seek immediate third party assistance.

7. When Your Counselor Has No Fresh Ideas: If your counseling sessions are boring, and the therapist is repeating what has been talked about previously, it may be time to terminate and seek out another helper. There is simply no reason for listening to repetition.

8. If You Are More Disturbed After The Sessions Than Before: Should you be more angry, depressed, or disappointed following a session than you were before, perhaps the technique used is not getting to the heart of your problem. Sometimes a professional criticizes you under the guise of good therapy. Robbing someone of their dignity and self-worth is certainly not helpful under any circumstance.

9. Suppose Your Counselor Is Selfish Or Inconsiderate: If your mental health worker becomes rude or displays poor manners consistently, you might want to reconsider your choice. Some such problems may be that the person is late to sessions, cutting sessions short, not returning phone calls, charging for missed appointments, or eliminating your date without notifying you. Be alert also for offensive character traits, such as belligerence, sarcasm, or impatience.

10. What If Your Counselor Will Not Discuss Your Concerns?: If the person refuses to deal with any problem areas mentioned above, or other dissatisfactions you might have, then you would have to question his or her adequacy as a counselor. Some therapists get so angered as to say, "get out". Do not take such abuse; this is a good time to follow the suggestion.

Points To Remember

1. <u>When coping with the uncomfortable, there are some general considerations to keep in mind:</u> Negative emotions can be a natural response. You can only control your own behavior, not that of others. Detrimental emotions, if not dealt with, can become intense and damaging.

2. <u>Victimization is self pity:</u> You can rise from thoughts of helplessness. You will find the effort worthwhile.

3. <u>Rejection is reality:</u> People often discriminate against the disabled. Such conduct is intolerable. You can and should recover. Do not be distraught. Try to cast out troublesome events from your mind.

4. <u>Anger is psychologically and physiologically destructive:</u> Control your temper. Analyze your response. React to only what is important.

5. <u>Hostility is anger acted out:</u> It may cause guilt, poor physical appearance, and jeopardize your welfare.

6. <u>Envy interferes with interpersonal relationships:</u> The individual who focuses on what is lost may become angry. This could be a hindrance to plans for the future.

7. <u>Fear can paralyze you:</u> Sometimes you must surrender and do the best you can in the situation.

8. <u>There are many reasons for anxiety:</u> These include confusion over alternatives or mistaken belief or desire. You should be open to opportunities but not unduly concerned with the outcome. Venture brings success and venture brings failure. Keep an open mind.

9. <u>Guilt serves no useful purpose:</u> Take steps to eliminate it.

10. <u>Don't become alienated:</u> View yourself as an equal with others. Mix and mingle. Allow people to know you.

11. <u>Identify the downward slide of depression early:</u> Deal with the condition as soon as possible.

12. <u>Avoid isolation and withdrawal:</u> Decide to attempt to overcome rather than succumb to circumstances.

13. <u>Consider these points when selecting or continuing with a counselor:</u>

    a.   Are you personally compatible?
    b.   Do your values conflict?
    c.   Is your counselor too impersonal?
    d.   Guard against hero worship

e. Does your counselor have "hang-ups"?

f. Some professionals want to control you.

g. Look for therapist with new ideas.

h. You should feel better after a session

i. Do not Tolerate an inconsiderate Counselor.

j. If the person will not discuss your doubts, or exchange ideas in regard to the subjects, then he or she is not being helpful.

Chapter 5

Shaping Your Positive Self-Image

What do you really think about yourself? Do you believe you are able to accomplish things despite your injuries, or do you view yourself as a "helpless cripple"? These are important questions because they determine your self image.

A negative self-image, cannot always be totally attributed to the individual. Those with whom we are closely associated will also impact the way we feel about ourselves. Neighbors, friends, teachers, a mother or father, and even counselors can have a profound influence on attitudes we develop. Yes, and helping professionals can unknowingly contribute to impairing the perception disabled persons have about their abilities.

Peter Dobbs, afflicted at birth, had difficulty maintaining an optimistic view of life. He tried to remain positive by reading such books as: Move Ahead With Possibility Thinking, Tough Times Don't Last, But Tough People Do, and The Power of Positive Thinking. He spent hours listening to cassette tape programs, such as, The Psychology of Winning. When thirty-five years of age, Peter was hospitalized because of a back injury, and he could thereafter no longer walk.

One day his father entered the bedroom, and the young man remarked, "Dad, I hate to say it, but the reality is, I might not walk anymore." His father, not knowing how to respond, said

"Peter, if you can't walk, you can't do anything." Depressed, the son burst into tears. "Get out of this room," he screamed.

After his father left the hospital, Peter became increasingly depressed and sought the help of a Freudian counselor. Contrary to the books and cassettes of a goal oriented psychiatrist, Dr. Roberts believed in not setting goals for oneself.

In accordance with this view, the doctor counseled Peter that his problem was wanting the impossible. "After all, you are handicapped. People don't expect too much out of you. Don't expect too much out of yourself." Dr. Roberts then said it was his personal aim to receive eighty percent return for only twenty percent. When Peter showed him the book: <u>Success is Never Ending — Failure is Never Final</u>, he laughed and responded, "With your condition, you should define success as merely having fun."

Peter became confused and angry. He had tried in the past to accomplish many difficult things; now he was being ridiculed for his ambition. He wondered what to believe. Should he give up, or should he keep on struggling to achieve goals despite his circumstances. He did not know and began to not even care. As a result, Peter began to just lay in bed, thinking about suicide. One afternoon, after lying in a dark room all day, Peter got up from his bed and in pain shifted his body into the wheelchair, entered the kitchen, took a knife from the drawer and stabbed himself.

As you can see from the previous example, it is of the utmost importance to consider the advice of people who believe in developing your potential to the fullest. There is also nothing worse than a "negative thinking professional." Learn how to identify such people and disassociate yourself from them.

Coping With Competition Constructively

Today, we live in a world of competition. The disabled, in order to achieve their highest potential, must usually labor side by side with others in the workplace. That adjustment should be easier due to better educational opportunities, accessibility to buildings, and other social improvements. In the past years, most students with impairments had been segregated into special schools. The trend now is to integrate as many individuals as possible into environments with their able-bodied peers.

How can such a person compete successfully? Here are four ways:

1. Welcome Competition: As was stated earlier, since we live in a world where most of the people are without limitations, we should learn to compete with them. Let's define what is meant by competition. One way to view this is to try deriving the same level of personal satisfaction from your occupation as others do. Is this possible? Certainly! I believe that handicapped persons can also experience happiness and a sense of achievement. Of course, a person paralyzed from the waist down could not run the fifty yard dash, but he or she may find other ways to succeed.

As an illustration, why can't someone in a wheelchair teach college? Of course they can. Mrs. McGrath, stricken with polio earlier in life, is doing this at Sacramento City College in Sacramento, California. So, don't sell yourself short.

Don't Measure Yourself By Others Standards: It is unwise to analyze others with the idea in mind of matching their accomplishments. We are all unique and therefore our aspirations and abilities are different. For instance, an able-bodied free-lance writer told his class that he was able to write between twenty and thirty magazine articles per month. When Mark, who had multiple sclerosis and worked at a slower rate, wanted to match the production rate of this veteran writer, the youth, a beginner, became frustrated. He worked much slower, and his expectations were unrealistic, since an amateur does not become a professional overnight.

Cope With Problems Positively: When you compete in any capacity, most certainly there are disadvantages. Some people who write and lecture on success may lead one to believe that reaching it is automatic if the person will think positively. Did you know those who prosper are also hindered? They certainly are. For an individual with injuries, this may be true. Difficulties could seem overwhelming and the mountains too high to climb. What should you do then? How do you surmount these obstacles?   First, it is helpful to remember there is no gain without pain, seldom success without stress, and that everything nice has a price.   In other words, the key to confronting the frustration of trying to be competitive is to learn ways of coping with the unexpected in a careful and deliberate manner. Here are eleven ideas you might find helpful in dealing with adversities.

1. Every Difficulty Has A Limited Life Span
Most problems, even the tough ones, linger only for a given time. You can learn to solve them and deal with the matter creatively. For example, Don Wells was born with a severe speech and mobility condition. As a high school student and continuing until his graduation with a B.A. degree from college, kept searching for a vocational goal. Guidance counselors were unable to help him. It was not until almost twenty years of trying, that Don founded a nonprofit organization to help others. As this illustration do show a difficulty may take days, weeks, months, and sometimes even years to overcome.

2. Everyone Has Problems: A patient once asked his psychiatrist, "Do you know where I can go to escape all my problems?" The doctor pointed out the door to the East Lawn Cemetery and muttered, "You can join the dearly departed." The point is that no one is free from trouble. Those who prosper know that trials will arise, but they believe some kind of answer can be found.

3. You Choose How Your Hardship Will Affect You:
When you stop to think about it, this principle applies well to those

with disabilities. No one wants to go through life with physical problems. It is a circumstance over which we sometimes have no control. However, one has the choice of how to react to it. You can take an affirmative view or continue to be angry and wallow in self-pity. You make the decision.

4. There Is A Negative And Positive Response To Every Problem: Since you can choose how to react to a situation, you can select either alternative. For instance, in John's younger years, able-bodied children often asked questions about his impairments. Of course, this reminded him of the reality of his injuries. Then a good thought came to his mind. Why not use his responses to teach others how to react when meeting someone disabled. Wouldn't this be a worthwhile service to mankind? He applied the idea whenever possible. Somehow, the instances of being noticed, and the continuous questions became less annoying. Taking this attitude made such occasions more bearable.

5. Don't Exaggerate Your Trouble: It has been said that one should "not make a mountain out of a molehill." Then why are we so inclined to do this? Many of us, at one time or another are guilty of exaggerating. During the stressful periods, we may view our circumstances as the worse possible. It is helpful to remember when these times arise, the matter could be more disturbing. Flying back from a trip to see his critically injured daughter, a father was crying because her leg had been amputated. Then he paused and realized that the girl's misfortune might have been more serious she could have died.

6. Don't Aggravate The Hardship: We have the option of either making our situation better or worse. It is often just a matter of mental attitude. Many of us can remember times in the past when we faced real challenges. Rather than taking decisive action as quickly as possible to find a solution, we sat bemoaning the fact there was a problem. This is unwise, since one can spend needless time and energy harboring negative emotions. It is more prudent to do something.

7. Don't Underestimate Your Adversary: While it is unwise to aggravate your ordeal, one should not underestimate it either. Troubles are real and ought not to be minimized. Disregarding that basic fact is to live in a dream world. While continuing to ignore the unpleasant, a person delays finding an answer or adjusting to the circumstance. So, it is not advisable to "play down" your concerns or your ability to cope with them.

8. Consider Various Options: Frequently when we have difficulty, we tend to "throw up our hands," retreat without meeting it head on. But wait a minute, this type of reaction does not solve anything. Instead, try thinking that you have options. What are they? One of the best ways to find out is to have a "brain storming" session. First, get yourself in a relaxed state of mind and give thought to various possibilities, then write them down. Next, choose the options that appeal to you and work to transform those into reality.

9. Every Circumstance Will Change You: Trials can make you either a bitter or a better person. Not having a vocational goal forced Bill to become creative and to begin his own home operated business, making him a stronger person. It also taught Bill the lessons of patience and perseverance. One can usually learn something from every activity when you keep an "open mind" and an affirmative attitude.

10. Adopt Constructive Attitudes Now: It is useless to hope that others will solve your unhappiness or to continue regretting that hardship has come your way. How should you begin? One way is by developing a possible solutions list. Write down the numbers one to ten and list at least that many ways of solving the unsolvable. With different insights at hand, you now have numerous ideas for approaching your problems in new and innovative ways.

11. Although Circumstances Cannot Be Altered, They Can Be Managed: Some things appear permanent and resistant to change. A young boy was hit by a car and is paralyzed from the neck down. He will never walk or use his arms again. What do you do when such conditions cannot be changed? The answer is modify your attitude. In the words of the Serenity Prayer, "God grant me the serenity to accept the things I cannot change, courage to change the things I can, and the wisdom to know the difference." Even in the darkest times, we all should strive to remain positive. That is the choice worth making.

Develop A Positive Self-Appraisal

Is it within one's capacity to develop a positive self-appraisal? After all, you are disabled. Should you be downcast? Absolutely not. You need to develop a worthy conception of yourself. Can You? Of course you can. Many limited people accomplished that.

One New Year's Eve, a van drove up to the site of a party. A side door was opened and a teenage lady in a wheelchair was lowered to the ground. She was pushed inside and everyone greeted Sue who had cerebral palsy. Despite being unable to control any of her limbs or speak, she had a radiant smile on her face. After having assistance removing her coat and getting comfortable, with a head stick, she pointed to the letters on a word board that spelled the sentence, "Where is the Coke?" Then she grinned appreciatively as a friend assisted her with drinking. Sue conversed with other guests all the while enjoying herself as she slowly constructed her sentences. pointing to one letter at a time. Even though severely impaired, a positive self-appraisal enabled her to have fun at the gathering.

Accept Yourself

Another word for acceptance is contentment. There is a "contentment principle" which is not new. In fact, the Apostle Paul in 61 AD, while in prison, wrote these words; "Not that I speak in regard to need, for I have learned in whatever state I am, to be content. I know how to live on almost nothing or with everything. Yes, even in the trying times, we can often profit from our experience.

Believe You Can Succeed

It is important for one to maintain a positive attitude. Someone might ask if this is attainable in a world where there seems to be so much rejection, discrimination and negative impasses to overcome. Where is the power to remain positive?

We all must have the faith to succeed, the belief that our status can be altered sometime, some way, some day. Just what is faith? One dictionary defines it as "complete trust or reliance." Although some among us may think that the able-bodied do not really give us an opportunity to prove our worth, one can still cope with these negative reactions and opinions by faith. Here are three methods of developing this assurance.

1. Believing Before Seeing: You have heard the phrase, "I must see it before I believe it." These two illustrations substantiate the opposite point of view. People said that Bob, confined to a wheelchair, would not progress further than special education classes, but he is beyond, as the recipient of a Master's Degree. Others snickered when he remarked that he wanted to write a book, but a year later that became a reality. These accomplishments proved that believing something might be possible, and sometimes can bring it to fulfillment.

2. Look For The good: Ignore the bad. As people who live with injury, there are many times when we have become indignant. Anger often surfaces when people tell us we cannot engage in certain activities because of our situation. This can be

FAILURES ARE

DETOURS

NOT

TERMINATIONS

most distressing until he or she accepts that one must look for the good while over ignoring the bad. It profits nothing to harbor resentment. We really shouldn't expect to fully understand our situation when others cannot. We might instead focus on the possibilities for our lives, rather than the agonies we face.

3. Self-Reliance: Some of the best progress one can make may result from turning inward and concentrating on being resourceful. Professional guidance can be invaluable, but as one college instructor at times would remark, "You have to learn to row your own boat."

Failure is Never Lasting

Many rehabilitation counselors have low expectations regarding the disabled. Karen Williams, a freshman in college had just recovered from brain damage due to an accident. Karen approached her counselor explaining that she wanted to be a teacher, and the response was "Don't you know you have multiple handicaps? Creative writing would be a good pasttime for you, out of the public view. No one likes to look at a cripple."

Both professional and nonprofessionals many times take a dim view of anyone limited. In many cases attitudes or prejudices against an individual are a greater hindrance against them than the person's physical status.

Trying Versus Not Trying: Many with impairments are highly motivated, but able-bodied individuals, when talking to those with impairments, use such phrases as, "lower your expectations," "your goals are unrealistic." or "It's impossible." Those statements when spoken are usually meant to be helpful but tend to discourage the individual. To put this in proper perspective, it is important to remember these facts. First, for anyone, having been injured or not, there are always risks. No venture is risk free. Second, if you don't try, of course you will not experience pleasure and satisfaction. No one accomplishes anything without an attempt. Third, if you try there is always a possibility you may succeed and prove your doubters wrong.

Never Be Frightened Of Failure: People sometimes withdraw for fear of failure. But, to fail really should not be of great concern or devastating. Of course, no one likes to fail, and we would all like to succeed. However, many great people have experienced reversals. English novelist, John Creasy received 753 rejections before he published 584 books. The Macy store failed seven times, then became successful. Babe Ruth struck out 1,330 times, but also hit 714 home runs. So you fail, then join that group of losers who kept on to become winners.

You Can Start Again: The wonderful news for those who have been defeated, is that you can begin again. Of course, nobody enjoys starting from ground zero and reconstructing a project that once had been established. But remember, you did it once. You can do it again. Keep trying, perhaps one day you will succeed. Quitters never do.

IF AT FIRST

YOU DON'T SUCCEED

TRY, TRY AGAIN!

Look For Opportunities

Some disadvantaged persons think that because of their injuries, they have no opportunities. For instance, if you are searching for a vocation, of course, the openings could be fewer, and the task of obtaining a job could be more involved. Don't surrender to defeat. Your desires might not be hopeless. Never say never. Here are four suggestions:

Analyze Personal Abilities: Examine your strengths not your weaknesses. As Dr. Karl B. Carlson, afflicted with cerebral palsy, stated in his autobiography, <u>BORN THAT WAY</u>, "Even the most hopelessly handicapped can be useful to society." For example, Diane, a quadriplegic with unintelligable speech, used a headstick to write articles for national magazines and earned an income from this activity.

DISCOVER YOUR INTERESTS: Just because someone with restrictions is able to do a task is no reason he or she should be doing so. For instance, Robert Williams, who had a communications impediment, enjoyed math but preferred to counsel disabled people. His college counselor asked, "Why don't you become a statistician?" "Even though I like math", Robert responded, "I desire working with people, and would not be happy working with numbers on a longterm basis." Remember, most of us are not successful doing what we dislike.

Dare To Be Different: Some individuals might want to look for non-traditional or out of the ordinary ways to accomplish their aims.   As an illustration, Jerry Williams, who was deaf, wanted to work as a Social Services Director.   No one would hire him.   After much frustration, he founded his own non-profit organization and is now working with other deaf people, busily and happily motivating them.

Never Stop Dreaming: David Murry was blinded in World War 11 when a shell exploded in his face.   He had a home on the edge of a lake and had always yearned to build a cabin cruiser, but how could he?   He found someone to tape record a book about boat building, then proceeded with construction. Having some assistance, David accomplished this task, and was gratified with his success.

Do Your Best

Some years ago Thomas J. Peters and Robert H. Waterman, Jr. wrote the book *In Search of excellence,* describing how leading companies prosper by maintaining high standards. Just as this is essential in the business world, it is vital in the lives of individuals.   Unfortunately, in the last decade of the twentieth century, many people have settled for a standard of mediocrity. A prime example is that in many communities, high schools are graduating students unable to read well or write fluently. This is tragic, but true.

However, each one of us, no matter how lowly the occupation should do our best. This is even more essential for someone disabled. To reach our fullest potential, we might also put forth a little extra effort. By so doing, you can make progress toward shaping a positive self-image.

Points To Remember

1. Don't Shy Away From Competition: You may be able to do more than you think.

2. Never Compare Yourself To Others: Be happy with what you can accomplish at any given time. Later you may be able to do more.

3. Cope With Difficulties Creatively: Remember these guide lines:

 a. Every problem has a certain life span.

 b. All people have difficulties.

 c. You select how hardships will affect you.

 d. There is a negative and a positive reaction to every trial.

 e. Never exaggerate your trouble.

 f. Be careful not to aggravate your circumstances.

 g. Consider various options.

 h. Every problem will change you.

 i. Take constructive action now.

 j. Consider which situations cannot be altered.

4. *Develop A Positive Self-Appraisal.* Consider your abilities.

5. *Accept Yourself:* Try to be content with your status.

6.*Believe You Can Succeed.* Keep in mind these points:

      a.   Have confidence in yourself.

      b.   Look for the good — ignore the bad.

      c.   Develop creativity.

7. Failure Is Never Lasting: By not trying, you surrender to failure. Wipe out the fear of failure, since many make mistakes. You can always try again.

8. Look For The Opportunities: Analyze personal abilities and interest. Dream creatively.

9. Have A Vision for Excellence: Set high standards. Put forth your best efforts.

Chapter 6

Develop The Courage To Try

As a child, Fred Morgan loved to ski. At age four, his parents taught him the sport and almost every weekend during the winter months the family was on the slopes. When he was twelve, he developed bone cancer in his left leg, and it had to be amputated. One day his mother walked into the hospital room, and he said to her, "I'm sure going to miss the slopes." She asked, Who said you had to? Haven't you heard about amputee skiing? "Yeah, I think so. Do you think I could learn?" He asked. His mother responded, "Are you willing to make the attempt?"

Someone once said that everything nice has a price. Courage is doing whatever it takes to accomplish something. As we start this chapter, let me pose two important questions: Do you have the inner strength to accomplish your heart's desire no matter how difficult it could be? Would you still try despite what others say and how slim the odds?

Forget The Past

Accept Your Present Condition: No matter if you were born with a disability or acquired one later in life, it is essential for you to accept yourself with all physical limitations. This is not easy, but is necessary. Be sure you have successfully completed all stages of adjustment and dealt with all negative emotion as discussed in earlier chapters.

Don't Look Back: It is understandable how someone could ponder happier times of yesterday, and wish that if only things were the way they were then. This is foolish. At such times, a person has a choice to make. Either one can live with regrets, which is like having "clouds over the sun" in your life, or one place the emotional pain in the background and try to derive the most joy as possible.

The Meaning Of Courage

Do you know the meaning of courage? One way of looking at this term, is to realize that every letter of the word stands for a principle that helps us to understand the concept better.

'C' Stands For Commitment: You are committed to something. It could be a religious belief, a goal you set for yourself, the "I'll make a difference" attitude, or physical rehabilitation. Whatever you choose, it gives you a purpose and direction for your life.

'O' Stands For Outgoing: Wallowing in self-pity or lying in bed all day bemoaning the fact you are disabled, indicates you are not part of the community. We have to keep trying to make the best of the situation. This happy person is not ashamed of his or her differences, but views them as challenges.

'U' Stands For Unwavering: When you have courage, you are unwavering in your determination that you can and will be of benefit to yourself and others no matter how uncertain the path is ahead. You make a promise that you will not give up no matter how dismal the circumstance. You are persistent in a desire to do your best to make the days as productive as possible.

'R' Stands For Reaching: Anyone who has courage is always reaching for new opportunities and consistently searches for ways to improve living. The individual wants to prepare as best he or she can for the chances that may arise later in life to work hard to make their ambitions come to pass.

'A' Stands For Anticipation: One famous, minister Dr. Robert A. Schuller, was quoted as telling his people, "Something good is going to happen to you today." This is the attitude handicapped persons with courage are determined to maintain. They expect that the best will happen to them, and work to bring that about. Such an individual awaits each day in anticipation of what is to come.

'G' Stands For Goodness: As was stated earlier, disabled people should learn to ignore the unpleasant, and direct their attention on the best that is around them. Of course, bad things do happen. Discrimination does exist. However, thinking only on the irritable things, clouds our minds and our focus is drawn away from the positive. So concentrate only on good things.

'E' Stands For Enthusiasm: A person who demonstrates courage has faith that somehow and some way things will turn out for the best. The individual is never too concerned about temporary setbacks because he or she expects to ultimately be a winner. Each morning when arising, there is excitement about the day that is beginning and the opportunities it holds.

You Need To Succeed

A handicapped person may wonder, and rightly so, "Why should someone keep trying in the face of insurmountable obstacles?" For instance, Debra, who had a severe speech problem, asked her therapist, "Why should I strive to improve when my rehabilitation counselor closed my case and said I was unemployable? In other words, no matter what I do I am not good enough."

Many disabled people want to succeed, get off government assistance, and want to gain employment. However, once they finish their education, they cannot find a job, because of their severe disabilities. When faced with this situation, how do you find the will to go on? Being limited, we really only have two options: to give up without exploring all the possibilities that could be open to us, or go forth with faith to meet and beat the challenges before us. To keep from experiencing a mood of depression, here are some reasons for desiring the will to try:

Self-Esteem: There is no other human value so essential as self-esteem, the feeling of being useful regardless of what others might think. Of course, there is some discrimination where many of the handicapped are concerned. The hopelessness, frustration and disappointment some physically limited feel is real and justified. However, ultimately it is not important how others value us but how we value ourselves. Surely, everyone wants friends and to be accepted. If we totally depend on those around us for our standard of worth, then we are impairing our own mental health.

Dignity: The person who keeps trying no matter how difficult the circumstances is continuing to hold onto some degree of dignity. Why is this so? One who is working is reaching out and trying to improve himself or herself. The desire to obtain personal objectives provides the individual with feelings of worth, pride and dignity.

Hope: It has been said that if you have hope, you can cope. Dreams of thoughts or accomplishments tend to keep one emotionally alive and striving. Do not allow your dreams to be dashed by negative thinking people; keep on trying although it may be a struggle. You can either solve the problems or learn to alter your mental attitude.

Motivation: Motivation is the force of desire. What keeps many enthused is that there is always a purpose for their existence. The opposite is also true. The person who often wakens in the morning without motivation, goes through the day aimlessly, feeling useless and bored.

Life is not a joy ride. You owe it to yourself, the Nation and the world to do the best you can every day. You also owe it to yourself to find your niche and the pleasure that it brings.

You Have Value

Some disabled people have the mistaken idea that they are worthless, and have little value. This is not true. If nothing else, you can be an encourager. In a world where there are so many who have low self-esteem, some will need an uplift. Let's examine the effects on a business man when he saw a young handicapped lady:

John Black, owner of a bait shop, was losing about $2,000 every month in his business, and had decided to close the doors. He loved what he was doing, but financially he could no longer continue.

One Sunday, while at church, he felt so depressed, until he noticed Pat, who was afflicted with cerebral palsy. She was lying in a wheelchair, and had a beaming smile on her face while raising her hands to praise the Lord...John thought to himself. "If that girl can be happy with those physical disabilities, surely, although I lost money, my problems pale in comparison to what she faces."

Pat was unaware of the effects on that man. Yes, all people have value. Sometimes we do not realize how much.

Replace 'I Can't' With "I Can"

The Real Meaning Of Those Negatives: Do you know the meaning of the words "I can't"? Often they are used incorrectly.

First, it is important to remember there are things many people cannot do physically because they lack the skill, strength or ability to do them. However, in many cases when people say "I can't", they really mean, "I will not." They are unwilling to give their best efforts to the task at hand.
They want to sit back and use their disability as a reason for not trying.

Use Good Judgement: Just because you can do something, doesn't mean you should do it. Investigate each opportunity closely. Ask such questions as: "Is this idea a project really worth my expenditure of time, energy and money? Am I physically able to master the task? Will I enjoy the activity I engage in?" Only by considering such matters closely, should you then decide if this is something you should pursue.

Seize Opportunities Affirmatively: Once you have considered the proposal and determined it is something you should pursue, do so confidently. By saying, "I can" you attempt to grasp the opportunity that lies before you. However, remember there is an element of risk in everything. Nothing is 100% sure. As was said in the last chapter, failure is never lasting. So when you are sure as to the merits of the idea, don't retreat, but move ahead affirmatively.

Your Scars Can Become Stars

We all feel hurt from time to time. Friends say things that have a negative impact on us. Those who do not like us can unleash ridicule in our direction. We even inflict emotional pain on ourselves by the way we think. We should learn how to turn our weaknesses into strengths. But how do we do that? Here are four ways:

1. Avoid Anger And Bitterness: When a person is hurt physically or emotionally, they may have a tendency to become angry and bitter. As was indicated in chapter one, anger can be detrimental to you psychologically. It clouds your mind so you cannot think clearly to solve the problems at hand.

Forget The Heartache: A young man who had been involved in an automobile crash, carried a picture of the crashed car he had been riding in. Frequently, he would take it from his wallet and describe the details of the accident to a friend.

One day during a counseling session, he took the picture out to show to Mr. Peters, who looked at it and then spoke. "Why don't you burn that photograph? It is making you sick."

If you keep remembering your hardships, doctors tell us this can cause a form of mental illness.

Decide To Be An "Overcomer": Determine, in fact decide, that you will be an "overcomer". Of course, the wounds are deep. The heartaches and disappointments could be many. However, you can do it. Make up your mind so you can and bounce back. Sometimes it may take days, weeks, or months. I've known disabled people who experience depression for almost a year before they can live life to the fullest again. Along with much persistence, effort and work, these people were able to pull themselves out of the mire of despair.

Learn From Your Hurts: If your misfortune involves a mistake, don't brood over the incident. Learn from it. There is no reason to agonize about what occurred yesterday, because the past is gone forever, and the future is yet to be. You cannot go back and undo what happened in the past. All you can hope to gain is to learn the lesson of what you did wrong, and try not to make the same errors again.

Benefit From Your Hurts: Instead of nursing your hurts, remembering every wrong you experienced learn to reverse them. Make this a project. Rather than mulling over the matter in your mind, think of creative ways to solve it.

A painful experience can make you more sensitive to the emotional needs of others. Only those who have had grief in their lives can really understand the sufferings of those around them.

Determination Makes The Difference

To succeed in life, there is nothing more important than developing strong determination. It is true, "Where there's a will, there's a way." Once you are aware of what you want in life, you must be willing to pay the price. This is never easy. So, how do you begin translating "pie in the sky thinking," into a force that will change your life?

Know What You Want: Set a goal. You and you alone can do this. It is advisable to generalize at first and not be too specific. For example; Don Williams, when he was a child, made a decision that he wanted to work with other impaired individuals. He made a commitment that the overriding purpose of his life was to serve others.

Be Flexible In Your Objectives: While it is helpful to set a goal and know what you want, give yourself some flexibility when establishing desired objectives. Using Don's experience as an example, he always stated that he wanted to assist the disabled. When people asked him how he was planning to do this, for lack of a better answer, and because he really did not know himself, he stated that he either wished to be a special education teacher or perhaps a counselor. Little did he know or imagine that he would establish Living Skills, Inc., and be the director of an organization he created. The point is that while it is well to have an overall goal, do not be too concerned if you are not certain of all the details. At times it is difficult to know exactly what a person wants to do in terms of a vocational career, because of his or limitations. In this instance, the individual should remain optimistic and pursue areas of greatest interest.

Beware Of Negative People: Probably one of the greatest obstacles to anyone's success is negative people with whom they come in contact. Worse yet, the "negative thinking expert" — the special education instructor who sets low goals for her students, the rehabilitation counselor who tells his client that he or she is unemployable. Friends could doubt our worth and those close to us may take a dim view of our potential. Parents, for the fear of failure, might dampen our desires. The best advice there is: "DON'T LISTEN TO SUCH ADVICE." There is an exception to every rule, and you could be that exception.

Keep On Believing: Keep believing in yourself and the goals you have set. Avoid negative persons who habitually belittle your desires. It could be that they are envious of your talents, or do not fully understand you. Be persistent. Be confident and press on with a winning attitude, since determination can make the difference.

Points To Remember

1. Forget The Past: Accept your present condition, and don't look back with regrets.

2. Each Letter Of The Word "Courage" Has A Meaning: Each letter stands for a concept.

> a.   "C" stands for Commitment
>
> b.   "O" stands for Outgoing
>
> c.   "U" stands for Unwavering
>
> d.   "R" stands for Reaching
>
> e.   "E" stands for Anticipation
>
> f.   "G" stands for Goodness
>
> g.   "E" stands for Enthusiasm

3. Everyone Needs To Feel That They Can Succeed: Four reasons are: It builds self-esteem, this provides dignity, hope is generated, and one develops motivation.

4. All Disabled People Have Value: Everyone can be an encourager.

5. Replace "I Can't" With "I Can": People who say "I can't" may mean they really don't want to. When making a decision to do something, use good judgement.

When a conclusion has been reached, seize the opportunity affirmatively.

6. Your Scars Can Become Stars: Avoid anger and bitterness. Forget past experiences and decide to be an overcomer. Learn from your hurts and benefit from your experience.

7. Determination Makes The Difference: Know what you want, be flexible in your objectives, beware of negative people, and keep on believing.

Chapter 7

Goals Despite Disability

Judy Morris, a paraplegic, had just graduated from high school and planned to attend a local community college in the fall. Many mornings, she would sit in her wheelchair with a forlorn look on her face.

One morning, her mother asked Judy, "What's wrong, dear? You seem so sad. Can I help you?" Judy responded, "At times, I feel so worthless. I really don't know why I'm here. I don't know what I want and I don't have any real direction in my life."

Many handicapped people feel this way. What is the reason? They simply don't have any goals for personal development. One of the reasons could be a fear they cannot achieve them. However, as we said in the last chapter, one must learn to replace the words, "I can't" with "I can."

Define Your Life Purpose

In order not to seem useless, everybody should develop a life purpose. This gives each one of us a reason for living, not just existing. Our plans can be as varied as the differences of individuals and can either be general or specific.

The General Variety: Often when a disabled student enters college, because of his or her limitations, it is difficult to identify a specific goal. This does not mean you have no reason for going to school. One aim could be to develop some personal interests. A social worker once told his client, "You go to school for learning, not a job." In many respects, he was correct.

The Specific Variety: Sometimes it is easier for a person to select a particular educational or vocational goal. For example; someone in a wheelchair could be a disc jockey, that is, if he or she had no speech defect. The important thing to remember in selecting a specific goal is that you are physically and mentally able to perform the work on the job once you are trained for it.

Low Aim Is A Shame

It is a waste of human potential that some limited people are not more aggressive, and are content to accept the status quo. They don't reach for a higher rung of the ladder, not expecting much out of life, so they never reap the rewards of success. This can have many devastating consequences. Here are four:

Apathy: Individuals without goals, and without a sense of direction, may tend to mope or go through the day unhappily. They may go to bed at night, saying to themselves, "What contribution have I made to the world today?" If this attitude is allowed to continue over an extended period of time, it can lead to a sense of futility and even depression.

Non Improvement: When you set no aims or objectives, you block the desire to excel. By not planning or having low goals, you are actually saying to yourself that you are not worth much and you wander through each day without any strides to improve yourself. Some elderly persons sitting in their rocking chairs, say, "If only I had done this or that, things would be different." Isn't that foolish? Why not do your best today, so you will have a better tomorrow and not be living with regrets.

Not Reaching Your Top Potential: If you never set goals and try to reach them, you will not discover your fullest potential. Others fear starting a venture because they are afraid of failure. As was stated in an earlier chapter, failure is nothing to be feared. Have more concern about the opportunities you may have missed. Consider this thought. Think of yourself as an athlete. Just as a high jumper raises the bar higher and higher until he misses, set your goals beyond what may seem possible now. Then reach for those lofty desires. Come on. You can do more than to think you can. Of course, you may have a setback. But don't be discouraged. Just try again.

The Joy of Winning: If you are always "putting yourself down", and having low aims, you may never experience the joy of winning. You could feel helpless, knowing that your life has no direction. We all need to acquire a sense of accomplishment and become aware of, and be grateful for, our special gifts and abilities. When recognizing these unique talents and making use of them, more of us can experience success. Having goals for personal achievement is one way of acquiring this satisfactory feeling.

NO MATTER

WHERE YOU ARE

REACH FOR A STAR

INSPIRATION
PLUS
MOTIVATION
PLUS
CAREFUL THOUGHT
PLUS
HARD WORK
EQUALS
SUCCESS

Think About Your Limitations

It is very important to be cognizant of both your limitations and capabilities. You must be careful to realistically accept your inabilities. A handicapped individual always should try to remain positive, but at the same time evaluate activities in terms of the restrictions imposed by a person's disability. Failure to do this can cause dire consequences. For example; Jack, born with cerebral palsy, visited a show where there were different business opportunities on display. After gathering information on various possibilities, he decided to purchase eleven vending machines. Several people including the company representative, explained reasons why managing this kind of business would be difficult for him to accomplish, but he would not heed the advice given him. As the day approached when the machines would arrive, and the installation was to be made, he became aware of problems. He decided to hire someone, but soon realized there was not enough money generating from the business to employ a helper. Sadly, after spending over $11,000, he had to dissolve the business venture.

What are some ways for you to know if you can succeed in an undertaking?

EVALUATE YOUR RESTRICTIONS: It is one thing to be positive, but take care not to go overboard. After all, you don't want to "bite off more than you can chew." Take time and carefully assess all troublesome tasks. Ask yourself how much you can do , and in what areas you will have difficulty performing the work involved. This is not easy to do. Why is this the case? It could be that basically some physically impaired people want to forget their limitations. It is almost as if they did not want them to exist or believe that as they go along, somehow things will be solved.

Not only should one consider if the venture is manageable, but think about the fatigue factor. Often it takes disabled persons a great deal longer to accomplish something than an able-bodied person. They must use considerably more effort while doing their work. For example; Bill operated a small business. He had to awaken at 4:30 AM, dress, groom, eat breakfast, and meet a specially equipped van to arrive at his office by 9:30 AM. Since he used a wheelchair, he was much slower. When he closed the business for the day, he would sometimes stay late and not be home until 11:00 PM. Bill then went to bed, only to arise the next morning to start the routine all over again. After weeks of this schedule, his health began to deteriorate.

Stress is another factor to consider in evaluating your inabilities. Bill's business was so hectic, and too many hours at work made him an emotional wreck. He became highly nervous and began to withdraw, simply because of the pressures this type of job placed on him.

Do A Task Analysis: Before you embark on any kind of chore consider the activities involved. Don't be too hasty. You want to make sure your idea is likely to be successful before you take the plunge. Let's see how this works. Jerry wanted to make money for a nonprofit organization by putting coin canisters in local businesses. He wanted to check the feasibility of this idea, so Jerry did a task analysis. The first thing to contemplate was transportation. Since he could not drive, he must use public busses. This would take too long, so initially he could see the idea was not a good one.

Calculating Your Cost: If you are thinking about a project that involves a great deal of money, be sure to determine the cost beforehand. Since many disabled persons find it difficult to gain employment, some may plan to go into business for themselves. The newspapers and magazines are filled with advertisements, promising big profits. There is one basic rule to remember: examine all claims before making an investment. Never forget, everything that glitters is not gold.

Finding The People Power: The first thing to keep in mind is whether you might feel your time and efforts would be better spent in another endeavor.

Finding Someone Dependable Takes Effort And Patience: To begin your search, here are a few suggestions. Talk to others who are handicapped in the community. Find out how they recruit help. Then contact various agencies that work with physically limited individuals. Often, they are high school, college or university students looking for part time employment who are willing to assume added responsibility.

When it is time to hire, you should make a careful choice. There are some things you may look for during the first interview and in the weeks the person begins working for you. Remember these guidelines:

1. When talking to the individual for the first time, ask yourself the following questions: Is his personality compatible with mine? Does it appear that he likes me, and do I like him?

2. Find out if he has a current drivers license and has automobile insurance.

3. Make sure to get character references.

4. After you hire an attendant, analyze his work habits. Does he or she follow instructions, or pretends, to understand them?

5. Is your help on time and does he do the job efficiently? Responsibility is important. After all, you are depending on this person for many of your basic needs.

Consider Your Talents

Why and how should you contemplate your talents? Is this really essential? It certainly is. Here are three valuable points to keep in mind.

Identify Your Interests: Did you ever stop to think about what you really like? What activities do you really perform well? This is something to which you should give considerable thought. Take out a sheet of paper and write them all down. Spend adequate time and do not overlook any. Each one could be useful in life, so try not to forget a single one.

Develop Each Attitude: If you have a number of talents, it is not advisable to develop just one or two, but the full range of your abilities. This is essential for everyone, but is particularly realistic for someone with physical limitations. Why is that true? Because after all, you are restricted. To compensate, you want to do better in as many ways as you can. This will give you a variety of things to do. You want skills you have strengthened, and interests you have cultivated. Also these can either be ways of passing your time with hobbies in the future, or lead to a vocational objective.

Reduction of Time: There is simply no point in trying to develop a skill for which you do not have a talent. For example; all the way through elementary and high school, Greg was not competent at math. Despite telling his counselor this, she still insisted that he take algebra and statistics. Greg took a first year algebra course, but failed it. The following summer he took the class again but really did not understand the concepts, even though he received a passing grade. Then one semester, Greg attempted to take second year algebra, but soon dropped the course because he was failing. He tried to take statistics without an algebra background, but that also proved disastrous. He spent a great deal of time in this effort for which he had no inclination.

Evaluate Your Desires

When determining your talents, it is important to evaluate your desires. What do you like to do? What can you accomplish well? Sometime, sit down and analyze yourself. Remember, no one is really good at something that they do not like to do. Did you know that according to some statistics, 80% of Americans dislike their jobs? This is not psychologically healthy. No wonder there are so many emotional break-downs. When you stop to think about it, there can be few things worse than spending your week doing something you detest intensely. So it is important to identify those things you really find pleasure in doing, to avoid becoming involved in activities you may not enjoy.

How Goals Produce Motivation

Why Objectives Are Necessary: Why are objectives necessary in a person's life? There are three good reasons. First; they provide some direction. The individual thinks he or she is accomplishing something. Secondly, goals produce a desire. The worker becomes interested in what is being done. Finally, this idea leads to enjoyment. When anyone is occupied with something they like, the hours, days, and weeks go by so quickly.

Make Your Aims Manageable: As was indicated earlier, be sure that the goals you set for yourself are manageable. "Don't bite off more than you can chew," because if you do, there might be adverse consequences. You could feel overwhelmed, and want to quit what you are doing. In turn, this will cause a defeatist attitude, and you may hesitate to try again.

Set a Realistic Time Frame: Be aware of the time involved to accomplish a task. Remember to realistically evaluate how long a certain activity will take. Never underestimate, but plan that the goal might actually take longer than you had originally anticipated. Then ask yourself; Are you willing to spend so many hours to reach your objective, or are you likely to quit before it is completed? Your answer will determine if you should pursue the project.

Consider Your Values

Why should you think about your values? What are values? One definition is anything you deem to be of overriding importance. Generally speaking, whatever you hold in highest regard should be taken into account when determining your selection. Let's look at these three examples.

Money: Some people place a high value on money. They want a great deal of it to purchase the nice things of life. For them, the first thing they ask when taking a job is: How much will I make? They want to accumulate great amounts of wealth, and so they center their life around this effort.

Prestige: Some people desire fame. They yearn for others to recognize them. Such a person wants to maintain a high profile. Some movie actors and actresses fall into this group. They want others to notice them. In so doing, thus boost their ego, and they feel good about themselves.

Service to Others: There are those who like to be of assistance to others. They want to see them develop their life and receive as much enjoyment as possible. Therefore, they will want to work with people. Many individuals who are retired spend a great deal of time helping others in need.

Goals And Resources

By now, you have seen the importance of direction in your life. Now it is time to ask yourself a question. Before you do, remember this important point: *Don't waste your life, yourself and others and make this world a better place.* Now, consider personal resources, abilities, values and talents. Set a goal that is obtainable, then start moving toward it.

Points To Remember

1. Define your life's purpose: This may be done in either general or specific terms.

2. Low aim is a shame: It produces apathy, non-improvement, and failure to experience the joy of winning.

3. You should take a careful look at your limitations and abilities: Determine what you can and cannot do.

4. Goals produce motivation: Some particular aims provide direction, desire and enjoyment of life.

5. Consider your talents: Identify them. Developing each aptitude will help you establish meaningful objectives.

6. Evaluate your desires: Know what is important to you.

Chapter 8

Projecting A Pleasing Personality

In the next four chapters of this book there will be a discussion of various aspects of relating to other people. So far, we have covered how we deal with our inner most feelings, and gain the correct perspective on our disabilities and life in general. However, none of us live in a world of isolation. We all must relate to others—friends, relatives, peers and strangers. We need to learn ways of dealing with our associates successfully.

Like Yourself

We have already mentioned the importance of a good self-image, regardless of the physical limitations, it can lead one to a happy, productive, and contented life. This is significant because without it, we can hinder our relationships.

Judy, who had contracted polio, felt very self-conscious about her disability. She didn't like anyone reminding her of the limitations she faced. One day she went to apply for a receptionist position at a real estate office. Mr. Brown, the manager, greeted her and asked, "Can I give you a hand? "No!," she snapped. "I am able." Mr. Brown had already made up his mind that he was not going to hire her even though she had good clerical skills. She was not at all diplomatic regarding her impairments. Her unkind response of not wanting to accept help could be detrimental and might turn some people away from doing business with the company. Such a response is definitely not advantageous.

As the illustration demonstrates, Caroline was uncomfortable because the gentleman had noticed her affliction. This became apparent to Mr. Brown and resulted in the young lady not being hired. Those who are limited and have learned to like themselves also know how to make others feel at ease in their presence.

Mike, who had cerebral palsy, was wheeling himself down the street in his manual wheelchair on a hot afternoon. It was quit a struggle. Suddenly, a man emerged from an office and asked, "Where are you going?" Mike answered, Down the street about a block. Could you use a push?'. The man asked. Mike responded, "Oh, you are so thoughtful. Yes, that would be helpful." Mike realized that at times he needed help, and at the same time made others happy by allowing them the opportunity to help." I'm really a slow poke without my electric chair," Mike joked.

When they reached the store and parted, Mike offered Mr. Davis $1.00 for assisting him. The man, Mr. Davis, responded, "I don't want money. Meeting someone with such a grateful attitude is payment enough."

Liking yourself can be a real plus in public relations. The contrary is also true. It is a magnetic or repelling force as illustrated with Judy's and Mike's encounters. Therefore, this is another reason for accepting your physical disabilities and revealing this fact in your interpersonal relationships.

Wear A Smile

A Common Perception: There is a common perception on the part of the general public, that it is at least unpleasant, if not unbearable, for someone in a wheelchair. Of course, this is untrue. It all depends on the chair-bound person's attitude. Nevertheless, this impression does exist.

Everyone Has Problems: Difficulty and hardships are not just confined to someone with physical impairments.

The factory worker who has just been laid off a job after fifteen years has a problem. How will he support himself and his family? A teenager on drugs has a problem. He or she has a habit that can lead to a life of crime and perhaps an early death. Such an addiction can place some in prisons, hospitals and a casket prematurely.

Widows have difficulty. They are mourning the death of their spouse. A loss through death is not easy to deal with, and the emotional situation can be a hardship.

Such a person needs to see someone smile. Maybe the individual could be you.

Why Laugh: Why should you try to laugh when you meet people? There are two good reasons. First, it says to the person that although you have limitations, you can still make yourself feel good about yourself. Secondly, it indicates to others that if you can be happy in your condition, one who is able-bodied can be happy also.

Put Other's Needs First

Some people have attitudes about life which are unacceptable—attitudes that repel others and hinder the limited one from getting the maximum enjoyment from life. This is the view of: "ME FIRST", 'SATISFYING MY DESIRES', or "BUILDING MYSELF UP AT THE EXPENSE OF OTHER PEOPLE." It often has adverse consequences and portrays the person in a dim light. For example, when Mr. Jones told Jerry, "Sorry, we can't hire you," Jerry responded, "You are discriminating against me. Don't you know that employers should hire a number of handicapped people? It seems you are a bigot." Needless to say, this insulting reply left a bad impression of Jerry in the mind of Mr. Jones.

By contrast, suppose you put other people's feelings and needs first while also being intent on pleasing them; this can be an asset. During a job interview with a computer firm, Larry, who was born with cerebral palsy and had an "A" average both in college mathematics and computer courses, told his prospective employer, "I know I have some disabilities.

If you hire me, I will do my best so your company can grow and prosper." His attitude helped him gain that job opportunity.

Make Words Consistent With Deeds

You should always make your words consistent with deeds. Why is this important? There are three good reasons:

To prove a common misconception wrong: Some people believe that most limited individuals are incompetent and therefore cannot be given responsibility. Of course, this perception is incorrect. You should make sure that your behavior matches your words. To paraphrase an old saying, one gesture means more than that which comes out of your mouth.

To prove people can count on you: When you say something, people usually depend on you until your actions prove otherwise. On occasion, if you don't fulfill your commitments in a timely manner, you can bring a great deal of inconvenience to another individual. By not honoring your word, you are giving the message that what you said you really did not mean, and that their involvement in the matter is of minimal consequence.

To prove you can be trusted: If a person cannot keep commitments with someone else, the individual cannot be trusted. It is that simple. Of course, there will be unforeseen circumstances whereby one fails to keep a commitment. However, anybody who continually does not keep promises loses the favor and respect of others.

Establish Dependable Relationships

Building friendly relationships with others is often difficult and could be classified as an art. Why is making good friends necessary? On the one hand, no man is an island; we all need other people. But also you don't desire having persons take advantage of you nor do you want to associate with those of low moral character. It has been said that "birds of a feather flock together." You wish others to judge you by the company you keep, but how do you relate to people in a positive way? We will be dealing with that in some depth later, but for now, here are five simple rules:

Be Kind: Make certain you are a friendly person. Most of us do not enjoy the company of one who complains. Learn to laugh and have a good time. Avoid profane language; it only makes you appear uncultured and although some may not be offended, others probably will be. Take an interest in people, and as was stated earlier, have a genuine concern; try to fulfill their needs.

Be Reasonable: In relationships, you should strive to be reasonable, even during times of disagreement. There are several reasons for doing this.

When you find that another is opposing you, welcome the opposition. Take time to consider his or her reasons for contradicting you. The individual could have some valid points. After all, it is better to have wounded feelings, than to make a costly mistake.

Distrust your first negative impressions of people. These often are wrong. Get to know the person before making a judgement; it might be an acquaintance you will eventually like.

When anyone begins talking, don't interrupt. Allow them to finish what they are saying. After all, it is not polite to obstruct a conversation. So let the talking continue. Who knows, you might learn something.

Be cognizant of the areas you have in common. Build on these strengths. In the process, you may want to compromise. Be open to new suggestions, and then closely evaluate them.

Admit your mistakes. When an associate proves your idea is not right, acknowledge your error. Nobody is always correct. Be willing to say, "You were right. I was wrong." Be aware of your imperfections and let others know that you are.

Be Frank: There are some people with whom you should disassociate. For example; a friend who expresses dissatisfaction and misery every time you phone him. This can depress, and may affect your emotional health. As was stated earlier, it is unwise to continue being in the company of negative people. If you encounter such a person, you might be honest and simply say, "When we are together, your unhappiness really bothers me, so I have decided for the sake of my own mental health, we can no longer maintain our companionship." Perhaps, the individual will not like this, but at least you have been honest and have given a reason why you do not wish to remain close friends.

Be Rigid: Some people may try to win back your friendship even though you have told them that you want to end the relationship. Be careful, your own mental health is at stake. Of course, you may want to forgive and resume associating, but first consider the situation. If you think it is best to break away—be firm, hold your position, and don't retreat.

Develop Compassion

What is compassion? One way to think about this is by letting each letter of the word stand for some aspect of this quality.

"C" stands for caring: You really care about that other person more than getting your own needs met. John Dunn wrote a poem in which he stated, "We need one another. Treat each man as a brother. Treat each man as a friend." Be concerned about others. Be happy when they are joyful; weep and extend a hand of mercy when they are in sorrow.

"O" stands for Openness: Be open to people's needs. Don't say to yourself there is really nothing I can do, and then turn your back and walk away. The question is not "Can I make a difference in this world?" but rather, "Do I really want to?" If we keep our eyes and ears open, we can always find ways to touch the lives of others.

"M" stands for minimizing differences: Previously, we talked about being reasonable, and preventing disagreements from becoming arguments. No one wants to create enemies, and repel individuals so they will withdraw from our presence. Instead, like a magnet, we want to attract people. One way of doing this is to minimize differences.

"P" stands for pleasing: We already discussed earlier in this chapter about why it is so important to try pleasing our associates. It is so vital. Many of us who are handicapped, have a "Give Me" attitude, thinking that just because we are disabled, the world owes us something. This is not acceptable. We should replace the "Give Me" spirit with the "I will give to others." mentality. In so doing, we can be of service to others.

"A" stands for apologize: Why is it so difficult to say, "I was wrong. You were right?" The reason is that most of us have a big ego. A good word for this is pride. A person who wants to be correct at the expense of honesty is a fool, because he would project a false image rather than tell the truth. The problem is that often such falsehoods are revealed and the person's character is stained.

"S" stands for saying nice things: Control your tongue. Words have power to build a person's well being or to cut another to the bone. This tremendous force can be used in one of three ways:

To Direct: The words we say have the power to change the lives of others every day. We all give advice. The question is what type of guidance are we giving? Here are three points to think about. First, do I really know the suggestions I am giving are worthwhile? Second, is there any possible way my ideas could harm the individual? Third, have I researched my advice adequately so that I know it really works?

To Destroy: Words have power for good or evil. To reveal the type of person you are; if you are swearing, gossiping or criticizing, it discloses your true character. A factory foreman once told one of his employees in a heated argument, "Your nothing but a dirtball." The foreman's supervisor called him into the office and reprimanded him, saying, "I don't ever want to hear you say such a thing again. All our employees have dignity, and you better learn how to preserve it.

To Delight: One of the most positive ways to use words is to make others happy. A cheerful joke or story can give another joy. What you say and how you say it, has the potential to lift a person from the pit of gloom to loftier feelings of peace, joy and happiness.

"S" stands for staying calm: The second "S" in the word stands for staying calm. No matter how rude people become, with ridiculing, swearing and being obnoxious, stay calm. This indicates that you really care despite the person's actions. Sometimes people use bizarre behavior to display their despair, but you know they are hurting, and you are there to help.

"I" stands for interest: Be really interested in people. Don't be so self-centered. Find out about their greatest hurts and their greatest joy. What would they like to do? How do they feel about critical issues? Why do they think a certain way? Be understanding. Show an interest in, and be sensitive to all those around you.

"O" stands for other's needs: People basically are self-centered, but this is the wrong way to be. We should be more oriented toward our fellowmen. Don't think about yourself first. Think of those close to you. You will be surprised at the difference this will make in your pleasure and theirs.

"N" stands for nothing but serving: The whole idea of compassion can be summed up in the word "serving". As we said before, you want to make people happy; see that their needs are met, console a weary heart. By taking your eyes off yourself, and focusing them on others, you will find real joy and happiness. **TRY IT!**

It Pays To Be Punctual

Did you ever hear the phrase, "Time is Money?" What does it really mean? Time is valuable. Nobody wants to wait. There are places to go and things to do. Have you ever waited for a doctor who was late for his appointment? It can be a bore and an inconvenience.

Likewise, respect the time of your friends and associates. When you make a date to be some place at a certain time, be there.

Never give yourself excuses. If the date is for 3:00 PM, try not to be one minute late. To avoid this, plan to arrive early. Some people value their time highly, and will respect you for being aware of that.

Mind Your Manners

There are many ways to be polite. Why is this a consideration? The answer is obvious. Along with other socially acceptable manners, you should remember two words:

Please: Never forget that just because you are disabled, the world doesn't owe you anything. Therefore, when making a request say, "please." Otherwise, what you are requesting, may sound like a demand, and you should not expect others to respond to such bold arrogance.

Thank you: Now that the person has done what you desired, demonstrate that you really are appreciative by saying, "thank you." A limited person should cultivate a number of people who will offer assistance when needed. By saying, "thank you," and showing gratitude, you are more likely to gain the help you need in the future.

Points To Remember

1. Like Yourself: People often form their opinion of you based on the view you have of yourself.

2. Wear A Smile: A smile attracts people, while a frown drives them away.

3. Put Others Needs First: Be of service to mankind.

4. Make Words Consistent With Deeds: Don't be irresponsible. Show people you can be trusted.

5. Establish Dependable Relationships: Be kind and reasonable, but hold firm to your convictions.

6. Develop Compassion: Each letter of the word has a meaning:

> a. "C" stands for caring
>
> b. "O" stands for openness
>
> c. "M" stands for minimizing differences
>
> d. "P" stands for pleasing
>
> e. "A" stands for apologizing

f.   "S" stands for saying nice things

g.   "S" stands for staying calm

h.   "I" stands for interest

i.   "O" stands for other's needs

j.   "N" stands for nothing but serving

7. Be Punctual: Keep scheduled appointments, and be on time.

8. Mind Your Manners: Say, "Please" and "Thank you." Show respect.

Chapter 9

Coping With Negative Stereotypes

What is a stereotype? One definition is a preconceived idea about someone or something. Unfortunately, society has some faulty misconceptions that originated in the past.

A Historic Perspective

Throughout history the physically impaired have had a difficult time being accepted and integrated into our society. Most recently, the term "exceptional" is used to identify such individuals. This was not always the case. Ideas about handicaps were linked to mysticism, spirits, and the occult; words were used such as atypical and deviant to describe those who were different. Over the years, people viewed others having limitations with curiosity and fear. One reason for such apprehension could be that some of us are unaware of the person's real problems, and thus tend to withdraw from the unknown. Prior to the 1800's there was little research done concerning those who had disabilities; they were placed in jails, poor houses, and mental institutions. There was little compassion for them or interest in their well-being.

According to William M. Cruickshank and G. Orville Johnson, the religious atmosphere in early colonial America did not help the cause of the less fortunate. One would think others might have been more understanding, but in many instances just the opposite was true. Historians have said, the basis for this thinking might be attributed to misinterpretations of biblical passages. The Bible states, "man was created in God's own image." According to this belief, man was to be perfect. Therefore, since some were not, they were relegated to positions of inferiority.

It was only in the early half of the nineteenth century that individuals such as Horace Mann and Samuel Gridley Howe worked with socially maladjusted children. Reverand Thomas Gallaudet pioneered work with deaf children. Between 1817 and 1850, some strides were made in behalf of the handicapped in America. A school for blind people was founded in Massachusetts; in New York City, an institute for the blind began operating in 1832, and the Perkins Institute was founded in 1829.

On the one hand there was progress. Still, many physically impaired were sent to residential facilities out of the mainstream of society. While attitudes have improved today, misinterpretation still exists that can be damaging to the self-esteem of those who are limited.

People Do Not Understand

Today, there are numerous faulty ideas about the injured that many people tend to believe. Fortunately, with every passing year, these views are being diminished, but there is much to do yet toward completely eliminating erroneous beliefs and opinions so prevalent among the masses. The following is a clarification of these.

All Disabled People Are Helpless: Some people think that some of us are useless, helpless, and have no value to ourselves or others.

Mrs. Brown and Mrs. Myers as they walked down the street, saw Bob who was driving his electric wheelchair while controlling the joystick with his chin. Mrs. Brown exclaimed, "It must be awful to feel totally worthless. I would dislike being in that man's position." Bob, overhearing the conversation spoke up, I do have some abilities. I volunteer and do counseling at a mental health center."

Many, despite their afflictions, do have skills that can help them lead a life of fulfillment and service to others.

The Disabled Are Unable To Care For Themselves: There are persons who think all those who are somewhat disadvantaged should be taken care of by others. This was the experience of Bill, born with spinal bifia.

One day, in the early morning hours, he called the paramedics, and was rushed to the hospital. When he arrived, the attending physician asked a surprising question, "What board and care home did you come from?" When Bill answered that he lived in an apartment by himself, the M.D. seemed astounded and shook his head in disbelief.

The Disabled Are Possessed With Evil Spirits: While this idea is not too prevalent today, in colonial times, people thought the less-able ones in the community were demon possessed. Some even believed that parents who gave birth to an exceptional child were being punished for something evil they may have done in the past.

The Disabled Have A Communicable Disease: Believe it or not, there are individuals who think some permanent injuries are contagious when they really are not. This was the experience of Mrs. Boyer, whose son, James, was born with cerebral palsy.

To help James socialize with children of his own age. This mother decided to take him visiting with a neighbor who had a child as old as James. Besides wanting her son to associate with able-bodied children, she also liked to compare his development with that of other youngsters in order to evaluate his progress in areas she hoped he might improve. A few minutes after Mrs. Cooper had invited them in, Mrs. Boyer sensed a coolness in her welcome and wondered if she had come at an inconvenient time, since Mrs. Cooper was busy cleaning. Mrs. Boyer attempted to be friendly. She seated James on the floor by her feet and began a conversation, "I thought our children might enjoy playing together. They need companionship."

Mrs. Cooper continued dusting, while closely observing her son, Billy who sat some distance from James. The youngster began to crawl toward James, but his mother, seeing this, snatched her boy off the floor and disappeared into a bedroom, sharply saying, "Nap time, Billy!"

When Mrs. Cooper returned, she began to question Mrs. Boyer. "What'sa matter with your son? What's it he's got?" "James was born with Cerebral Palsy, but his condition is not contagious." Mrs. Boyer was feeling really uncomfortable, trying to convince her neighbor of this fact. "I'm not so sure," Mrs. Cooper skeptically replied. "There are so many thing that are catchin' and people keep always goin' around carryin' them. A person has gotta be careful."

Mrs., Boyer decided it was useless to explain that her son did not have a communicable disease and was shocked to think some people are reluctant to accept knowledge of the condition when advised.

The Disabled Are Emotionally Different: Individuals often believe the disadvantaged have a range of different emotional patterns, because they have bodily limitations.

Michael Peter, who uses a wheelchair, was lecturing before a class, and a student asked him the question, "I bet you get very angry and depressed about being handicapped?" "Oh no!," Michael responded. "I have learned to cope with it, just like able-bodied people deal with their hardships."

He has a point. Whether a person has been injured or not, we all have frustrations and must learn to adjust to them.

All disabled People Are Suffering: There are some who have a notion that the limited are suffering both emotionally and physically. That does not apply in all cases. As previously stated, many of those with physical impairments learn to have a wholesome attitude toward their situations. In terms of suffering, a person may or may not be in pain. This depends on their condition. However, while one who is learning to accept his or her circumstances, while the body may hurt, but the individual can often deal with it in a constructive way.

All Disabled People Are Unloving And Unfriendly:
There are able-bodied people who believe that the less fortunate
become so involved in their own problems, and are not concerned
with the needs of others. This could be true at times, but it is
certainly not valid in all instances. Some having limitations are
very concerned with improving social conditions especially for
this minority group.

All Disabled People Are Financially Independent: A
segment of our society think that most disadvantaged receive
government assistance. That may be a fact, but many physically
injured people want to work. In recent years, such agencies as the
Department of Rehabilitation have placed a greater emphasis on
finding occupations for the severely limited. Special problems
have been devised to aid with those employment needs. Many
disabled want a helping hand at finding work, not a government
handout.

Results Of Stereotypes

We covered just a minimum of the misconceptions that
some people have about handicapped individuals. How do such
attitudes negatively impact society? There are many ways, but
here are just three: First, it makes it more difficult for the able-
bodied and the afflicted to have a meaningful association. There
is fear on the part of many about how to relate to the one who is
different. Also, the injured have apprehensions as to the possibility of rejection. Secondly, negative stereotypes lessen the chances
that challenged people can make a significant contribution to
society. Thirdly, such views hinder the person's ability to reach
his or her full potential.

Therefore, such erroneous thinking has no constructive social value for anyone. Consequently, we need to change our reaction toward those who have such ideas, and then go about trying to educate them as to the abilities that we with disabling problems do possess.

Reactions To Stereotypes

There are two typical emotional reactions less fortunate persons could have to such treatment—anger and/or depression.

Anger: As handicapped people, we could say to ourselves, "Why must I be the brunt of such ignorance. It just isn't fair." Of course, it's not. Who said life treated everybody equally? Certainly, an individual who anticipates equality in all matters has unrealistic ideals. In chapter three, the question was asked: "Does anger really pay"? If anger is used in the wrong way, the answer is clearly "No."

How do you deal with the anger resulting from the misunderstandings of others? Remember these two important things. Anger can be destructive. It can rob you of the joys of life. Anger can be employed constructively to alter a circumstance. If this emotion is used in a positive way to bring social change peacefully, then it has accomplished something.

Depression: It is easy to feel depressed when you are the object of discrimination. Feelings of victimization and rejection might also result. However, never forget when you have a "pity party," no one will come, and if someone does, they more than likely won't stay very long. So what do you do? Sure you were hurt, but you have only one positive alternative: Pick up the pieces and move on.

Adjust Your Attitude

As was alluded to earlier, we must change our attitudes toward those who discriminate against us. Discrimination is wrong, just as slavery was wrong. However, there are two important factors to consider. One is that although you can try educating the public about attitudes regarding the injured, ultimately no one can change another's behavior. Also, don't forget that you ought not to allow anyone to determine the view you have of yourself. It does not really matter much what people think or say about you, it is how you perceive the situation. Negative messages will not harm you as long as you don't allow yourself to be devastated by them.

Attempt To Change Other's Views

If we are to eliminate negative thinking concerning the disabled in our society, each one of us must take action to change the misconceptions of those with whom we contact. How do we do this? There are a number of ways and here are some: Don't be intimidated by an associate. Just because one is able-bodied does not mean he or she is better than you. Next, if the individual has some mistaken ideas about you, make known your feelings.

Finally, do a little educating about impairments. Sometimes when people get to know someone with defects, their wrongful conceptions are altered and they value the relationship.

Demonstrate Your Abilities

A vocational Rehabilitation counselor once told a client, "You must prove yourself." These may sound like strong words, but they are for the most part, factual.

One of the misinterpretations is that the less fortunate are unqualified to do much of anything. Of course, this is not true, but often the afflicted must try a bit harder and demonstrate abilities in order that people might realize that somebody limited is capable of doing the task.

Make Others Comfortable Around You

How do you make people comfortable in your presence? This is a good question, since it is one of the ways you can help break down some of the negative impressions the able-bodied have toward those in your situation. There are numerous ways of doing this, but here are just four:

1. Don't Focus On Yourself: Nobody appreciates hearing a sad story about how bad life has been for you. Instead, try to be a pleasant, warm, gracious individual.

2. Be Interested In The Needs Of Others: How can you help them and lighten their burden?

3. Never Worry About How Much You Can Gain From Life: Instead, give of your time, talents and money to help those in needy circumstances.

4. Cultivate A Sense Of Humor: Stop taking life so seriously and learn to laugh.

Points To Remember

1. <u>In the early days of this Nation, disabled people were not treated well:</u> There was much fear and curiosity among the general population concerning them.

2. <u>Today many stereotypes still exist.</u>

    a. All handicapped people are helpless.

    b. The physically impaired are not intelligent.

    c. Those with impediments can never progress.

    d. The limited cannot care for themselves.

    e. Someone with afflictions is possessed with evil spirits.

    f. A person who is not able-bodied may have a communicable disease.

    g. Disadvantaged individuals are emotionally different.

    h. People with physical problems are always suffering.

    i. Anyone injured is unloving and unfriendly.

    j. The less fortunate are financially dependent

3. There are results of stereotypes: These harm both society and relationships between the able-bodied and disabled.

4. When discrimination is apparent, two typical reactions do exist: These include anger and depression.

5. You must alter your mental attitude: Try not to allow actions and remarks by some to affect you emotionally.

6. Demonstrate your abilities: Allow people to know you.

7. Make individuals comfortable in your presence: Don't focus on yourself. Be interested in other's needs. Give of your time and talents to mankind. Cultivate a sense of humor.

Chapter 10

Reacting To The Taunts And Stares

"Hey Niagara, your wettin' your shirt," shouted Buddy Tracy, a red-haired, freckled-faced bully, during the noon lunch period. "Hey you guys! Look at James! The way he walks, he looks like he had beer for breakfast! Let's tell the teacher." Mimicking his walk, Buddy paraded around the school-yard.

James, an eighth-grade student with cerebral palsy, took out his handkerchief to wipe away the saliva that was dripping from his chin. For a moment, he stood still, tears running down his face, then James raised his arm, and grabbed him.

"You fool," he yelled. "Leave me alone! Stop it!" Get your hands off of me," Buddy screamed. A teacher came over and stopped the fight. James seething with anger, sobbed, "Why must I be the object of such taunts and stares? Why am I the object of jokes and ridicule? Why must I withstand mockery, giggles and jeers?"

Such abuse can be quite cutting. It reminds us we are different, discriminated against, and others view us as objects of scorn or helplessness. This can have a devastating effect on our self-esteem. Nevertheless, this is a reality, and all of us should learn ways to cope with these uncomfortable situations.

Understanding The Problem

In order to cope with such circumstances in the best way, disabled individuals might first want to consider reasons for this type of behavior.

Adults React Negatively

Sometimes adults react negatively to people with afflictions and are not good role models for children. One study indicates this is true; Gerd Jensen and Otto Ester, two German psychologists, found that 73% of the subjects in a survey, felt that the handicapped should be kept in institutions away from the general public.

While attitudes are slowly changing, many people still don't know how to act when coming into contact with those having physical impairments. For instance, Mrs. Boyer went shopping with her fifteen-year old son, Willie, who had an abnormally large head and used a wheelchair. An elderly woman approached and asked, "What's wrong with your boy? Does he have water on the brain?" Willie, whose hearing was not defective, quickly responded, "Lady, — I have muscular dystrophy. My head is not completely filled with water, because I have an IQ of 120."

The sad fact is that when Jensen and Ester interviewed 1,060 adults, they found that 90% did not know how to conduct themselves in the presence of injured people. Obviously, this same group probably would never explain a condition of injury to their children.

Other adults are more understanding, but still find it difficult to answer their children's questions dealing with this matter. Since parents often feel unprepared to respond, the query is simply ignored. One such happening occurred when Mary Jo, a teenage polio victim, hopped down the aisle of a supermarket on crutches. Five-year old Jimmy stared at her, watching every step. Finally, he asked, "Why do you walk with those things?" His mother grabbed him, reprimanding her son sharply, "Shh.....Shh.....Shhh....Don't stare—I'll tell you later!" She pulled him away without ever discussing Mary Jo's handicap.

This is a common incident. When such a situation arises, often a parent has the misconception they should not mention a disability in the presence of the person. However, although nothing is said, there is communication. Because of this silence, the adult could be giving a message the able-bodied youngster might interpret as: there is something bizarre or strange about the individual that mother or father would prefer not to talk about.

Motivations Of Non-Disabled Children

Why do some youngsters ask questions, taunt, or stare at someone obviously different? Because of the negative parental influences previously discussed, the child upon seeing a disabled person may conduct himself or herself either by asking questions or by caricaturing them. To help you respond appropriately and not feel angered, you should try and understand what motivates the able-bodied boy or girl to react in this manner.

Asking Questions: A youth may approach you and ask, "Why do you walk like that? Why do you sit in a chair on wheels? Why do you talk so funny?" Of course, many of us do not appreciate others reminding us of our handicaps, especially in public. However, in such instances, by having a knowing and forgiving attitude, we can avoid negative emotional reactions. Those of us who are physically challenged should remember that in some cases, a young person is just exploring the world and perhaps has never seen anyone with injuries. For instance, this was the case with Joey, a five-year-old boy.

One day he and his mother went to the zoo, where Joey saw Lisa, a blind college student. "Mommy look. That lady is using a cane, "Why Mommy, why?" She replied, "Never mind. Be quiet!" Joey was insistent, "But mommy, that lady's using a cane and bumping into things". "It's not nice to stare at people. Come on, lets go look at the animals."

Joey hung back as his mother started walking away. Lisa, hearing Joey's questions, went over to him, "Hey Joey, want to know why I use a cane?" Shy, but curious, Joey answered, "Yeah. Why do you?" She explained, "When I was born I couldn't see. I don't know exactly why. I can do most anything anybody else can do. I use this cane to know where I'm going and if there is anything in front of me." Joey asked, "Will you ever see?" She replied, "I don't know. Perhaps someday."

Lisa had a good mental attitude when Joey inquired about her use of a cane, and realized he was just trying to find a reason for her condition. Being able to cope during such moments can also help improve your self-image. The real feeling you have toward being limited as well as providing a meaningful experience for the able-bodied person.

Accepting Disability

Five years ago, doctors discovered bone cancer in Amy's left leg and amputated the limb at the hip. At age fifteen, she had cultivated a more cheerful outlook on life. She had learned to accept the loss of her leg and to overcome feelings of being self-conscious because of the surgery.

One evening, Mrs. Coombs asked Amy if she would spend a few hours with Susie, her eight-year old daughter. After Susie's mother left, the girls were playing on the floor when the telephone rang. Since Amy's crutches lay across the room, she hopped to the phone and answered it. Susie followed, also hopping. She then asked, "Why do you only have one leg?" Momentarily, Amy felt somewhat stunned as she recalled the day when she awakened from the operation, picked up the blanket covering her, looked underneath, and saw her left leg had been removed. However, she knew Susie was inquisitive about her, so Amy attempted to explain.

"When I was younger, I was very sick. My leg became infected with germs, and the doctor had to take it off." Susie asked, "Why?" Amy replied, "So the rest of my body would not be sick, and I could live." Susie then said, "Oh, ok, now let's play a game."

The explanation satisfied Susie and no more was said. After Mrs. Coombs returned and had taken her daughter home, Amy lay in bed, thinking about the explanation she had given to her friend; it seemed not to affect their relationship in the least.

Inappropriate Behavior: There are many reasons why youngsters might ridicule someone with impairments. In fact, the list is endless, and unless a person would know the circumstances of a particular situation, it is difficult to pinpoint the exact cause for the behavior. However, here are five possible motives, any one of which could be a factor, depending on the incident.

First of all, the young, especially when under the age of five or six usually do not intentionally hurt the person they encounter. The child just might be curious, yet the mannerisms and tone of voice could indicate purposely taunting.

Shortly after Donna and her five-year-old-son Ricky moved into a new neighborhood, they were sitting on their front lawn one evening when Ricky stood up, pointed his finger to the driveway of the adjoining property, and said loudly, "Look at that boy in the chair! Mommy, is he lazy?" Ten-year old James, paralyzed from the waist down, heard the remark and slowly wheeled himself into the house. When inside, the youth called out, "That boy laughed at me!" "Cool it," responded his mother. "Stop being so sensitive. Come into the kitchen and have a snack."

While sitting at the table, munching on a cookie, the doorbell rang, "I'll get it," James said, moving himself across the room and opening the door. There stood Donna and Ricky. "I want to talk with you," Donna softly uttered while her son's eyes filled with tears. "Ricky has never before seen an injured person in a wheelchair and was asking about you. When I explained to him that you undoubtedly were disabled, he was so concerned and wanted to meet you." Then Ricky spoke, "I'm sorry, I didn't mean to hurt you. I'd like for you to be my friend." James felt humiliated, because he had misunderstood Ricky's remarks as malicious when they were only statements of curiosity.

As alluded to earlier, a second reason children stare and harass those with handicaps is that they might perceive the impaired person as acting different. Possibly, their parents have not yet had an occasion to explain to them that some people , because of an unfortunate occurrence need special equipment and so they appear unlike others. As a result, children coming in contact with someone in a wheelchair could gaze intently or even ask probing questions.

One example involved five-year-old Gerald who was enjoying the county fair. As he stood near a booth watching a clowns performance, he also saw Eva limping along on crutches and wearing braces. He left the clown sideshow and followed her, wondering to himself, "Why is she wearing those funny shoes with metal rods. They must not feel good, and why does she lean on those sticks. They seem to slow her gait."

Then, Gerald called out loudly, making sure Eva would hear him. "Where did you get those funny sticks?" Eva, feeling self-conscious, looked over her shoulder at Gerald and did not respond. He continued following her for some time, but soon lost Eva in the crowd. However, Gerald thought about her throughout the day, and wondered why she needed support to walk.

Thirdly, sometimes children are "morbidly curious" about those who seem to have had some misfortune before, during or after birth. The best description of this mentality is to compare it with the attitudes during the 1600's when American colonists put so-called ""witches" in stockades and stoned them.

During that time, it was widely believed that individuals were created in the perfect image of God, and anyone having physical defects could be possessed with Satan, the devil, or evil, and should be punished. For instance, early records left by commissioners of poor houses and visitors to mental hospitals implied that persons with epilepsy and other impairments were chained to stakes outside the buildings. Unfortunately, just as those with such ideas threw stones at witches in stockades and bound the disabled to stakes in courtyards,, some youth view the limited as odd or funny, and will ridicule them.

A fourth point to remember is that children and teenagers frequently delight in "showing off" to their peers. One way of doing this, while also demonstrating their power, is by harassing others who, in their opinion, are not able to defend themselves against verbal attacks. A good illustration was given at the beginning of this chapter as to Buddy's treatment of James during the noon lunch period. Juveniles with behavior problems often want to build their ego at the expense of someone whom they come in contact with.

Finally, some youth are more understanding when younger, but as an adolescent, may want to disassociate themselves from a disabled friend, thinking the image they hope to present to their peers will be more impressionable. The experience of John, born with cerebral palsy clarifies this point.

For several years, Kate visited John's home almost daily. They had become good friends and spent many pleasurable hours together, watching TV, playing games and going to movies. When Kate began dating, the relationship changed. Feeling lonely one morning, John decided to walk down the road to Kate's house and visit her. Kate saw him coming into the driveway—his body awkwardly bent to the right with his left arm raised upward to balance himself. When he neared the house, she ran out to meet him.

"Don't come in!", she blurted out. "We're having a party, and my boyfriend, Tom, is here. Anyway, you are a mess. Don't you know you are slobbering; the front of your pants is all wet. Go away! You would embarrass me!" John turned and sadly walked home, feeling humiliated and wondering why his long-time friend had treated him in such an adverse way.

Watch Your Emotional Reactions

As a handicapped person, how do you respond to questions and ridicule. Before confronting other people who have been disrespectful and abusive, it is important to examine your own emotional condition. Of course, these reminders are psychologically painful. No one wants to be singled out as odd or different; nevertheless, these incidents happen. So let us discuss some ways individuals can deal with these situations.

Inquiry

Some with bodily injuries respond to questions in different ways. A person may welcome them and answer positively, hoping to educate others about the nature of their condition. Gary Kline, a graduate student with cerebral palsy, states, "I'm flattered when people ask about my physical limitations. It gives me an opportunity to show them I have intelligence despite my speech and mobility impairments."

Others give the impression they are offended. There could be many reasons for this. Here are two possibilities. First, such inquiry can be an unpleasant reminder that the person is afflicted in certain ways. Some people are humiliated at the mention of their condition, since they want to be accepted as "normal." Consequently, these questions only serve to make them more aware of something they are trying to forget. Secondly, depending on the circumstance, the inquiry can be socially humiliating. For instance, if a child asks a woman in a store, "Why do you sit in a chair on wheels?" Other shoppers may look up and observe the situation. As a result one may then be the center of attention.

Ridicule

Ridicule can have the same affect as inquiry does, since it reminds one of his or her circumstances and may result in emotional distress and be socially embarrassing. However, even more importantly such behavior can lower the self-image, while also in some cases causes one to become angry. Now let's consider these two types of responses in more detail. Such remarks can have a negative affect on someone's attitude about themselves. This is true since nobody likes to be the brunt of cruel jokes and such behavior can only cause people to question their feeling of adequacy.

Many people, especially children, have difficulty maintaining positive self-esteem. When others ridicule them, this only adds to the individual's perception of himself and his abilities. Some who are limited may also become angered due to being taunted. They could develop the tendency to believe that the able-bodied are prejudiced against them, and develop a hostile and negative attitude which could alter relationships.

Expect Unfair Treatment

We live in an age where there is a quest for equal rights. Everyone wants nondiscrimination and to be treated fairly in all events. Many of us believe in equal rights and are emotionally crushed when people treat us with disrespect.

Let's stop living on Cloud Nine, Begin to expect unfair treatment and recognize that all people are imperfect. Some will not respond to you with dignity and will shun you. Instead, react negatively, remembering that all people will not like you and don't delude yourself into thinking otherwise.

But you don't have to keep experiencing such emotional pain. Just change your attitude, begin to expect unfair treatment. Some will not respond to you with dignity. Some will even shun you. Never allow yourself to be mortally wounded. All people will not like you. Don't be deluded otherwise.

Methods Of Responding

What are some of the best and constructive ways to deal with questions about yourself, stares, taunts, and ridicule. Here are some ideas:

Questions: Young children, teenagers, and adults may ask questions about someone's handicap. Therefore, it is important first of all to accept such inquiry as a natural part of your life and not be offended by it. If the person has really come to terms with his or her limitations, such questions will not have an adverse impact. Dr. William Rader, a nationally known psychiatrist, pointed out that if a physically challenged person really has it "all together" about who he or she is, anyone with whom he comes in contact will be more comfortable in their presence.

Secondly, respond to questions promptly. As Dr. Rader states: "The matter should be handled at the moment, so there isn't suspicion or anxiety arising from it." Be forthright in your response.

Jack, a veteran paralyzed from the waist down, sat in a wheelchair on the front lawn. Mike and David, were playing hide-and-seek across the street. When they saw Jack, they came over to where he was sitting, and Mike asked, "Why do you sit in that funny chair?" I noticed you wheeling yourself around," added David. "Can't you walk? I was shot in the spine when I went to war, "Jack explained. "The doctor removed the bullet, but now I must use a wheelchair to get around."

Satisfied, Mike and David asked no more questions and went back to their game. Thirdly, with young children, use simple language they can understand. Bobby, four-years old, stopped a man on the street and asked, "Why do you walk that way?" "Son, I was hurt." This brief response satisfied Bobby.

Fourthly, you can, if you wish, explain the medical aspects of your disability. Six-year-old Danny walked up to Shelly, who was sitting in her wheelchair. "Why can't you walk?" "Because when I was born, my spine, the big bone in my back, was not formed properly. I have an affliction called Spina Bifida."

Fifthly, try cultivating a sense of humor. If an individual can take a joke, his or her peers will feel more at ease. In a department store, seven-year old Jeff stopped in front of Don, who wore a hearing aid and stared up at him, and asked, "What's that tiny box and that book in your shirt? I can't hear too well," Don replied. "This helps me hear. I call it my radar equipment."

This man's funny remark, helped explain his hearing loss. Many times these confrontations seem awkward, but a joke is a good response to calm the tension during the interaction. Without being serious, he got his message across.

Lastly, assist parents in responding to questions about your disability. Instead of feeling self-conscious, help them answer the inquiry.

Michael and his father walked into a supermarket. Michael pulled back when he saw a man with a hook for his hand," and asked his father, "Why does that man have a hook?" While his father hesitated, the amputee walked up to the father and son, then spoke, "When I was younger, I caught my hand in a machine at the factory where I worked. The nerves and muscles were damaged and the doctor removed part of the arm, replacing it with an artificial one. It's attached with a strap around my shoulder behind my back. I can pick up money and even light a match." He showed Michael how his hand worked.

The youth seemed less apprehensive, since he could now understand the reason for the man using a hook. Later, at home, Michael told his mother, "You know there are many different people in the world, but they are nice."

Stares And Taunts: Questions are sometimes difficult enough to cope with, but staring and especially taunts, can be even more disturbing, since there is most always evil intent involved. Of course, adults also discriminate against adults, and this will be dealt with in a later chapter; but now let's focus our attention on ridicule of children and teenagers. Following are a few suggestions you may find helpful:

1. When someone makes jokes, mimics, or laughs at you, one of the worse things you can do is to show anger. There are three good reasons. First, the disabled person might become injured if there is a battle. Second, if the one responsible for the incident is hoping to annoy his target, and you become enraged, this only helps the instigator of the mischief achieve his goal.

Lastly, anger invites the prankster to keep brow-beating the victim who may be unable to control his or her temper and bodily, movements, thus causing the disadvantaged movements, thus causing the disadvantaged participant more physical agitation.

Avoid Self-Pity And Depression: In chapter four, we discussed at some length about how to cope with negative emotions. In relation to taunts and stares, the same principles apply. However, above all remember that you should determine your own self-worth. If you have worked hard, no matter the amount of ridicule you face, you can hold your head high knowing that even though you are at times challenged, you still can make a contribution to society.

Overlook Ridicule: Some people with impairments can confront the person who is abusing them in a positive way and explain how they feel. Others cannot, because they feel too devastated. One can choose to just walk away and avoid responding. Sometimes, doing nothing is better than engaging in inappropriate behavior.

Deal With Name Calling: Some children and teenagers will call disabled people names. Here is how one young man with cerebral palsy dealt with the situation:

John lived in an apartment, and next door was home for five-year-old Jimmy, five-year old Danny, and six-year old Mark. When they saw John, they would giggle and say, "Hey—Funny Man."

One day when John was outside, Mark yelled, "Hey— Funny Man. What are your doing?" John wheeled himself over to where the boys were playing, frowned, and glared into the eyes of Mark. In an authoritarian voice, he snapped at Mark, "My name is not Funny Man! Don't call me that! It's John! Remember that!" Scared to death, Mark meekly answered, "Yes, John." After this incident, these three boys never called John "Funny Man" again.

Please Don't Hurt Me: Judy, a sixth-grade student confined to a wheelchair, had just been integrated into a school with able-bodied students. One day, Martha hollered at Judy, "Hey girl! Are you lazy? Get up and walk." Judy burst into tears. Martha walked up to her and "It's Halloween. I was just having fun. Of course, that chair is part of your costume. Why are you crying? What's wrong?" "Oh, I wish this was just part of my costume," Judy sobbed, "You do not understand, this is not fake. I can't even stand, much less walk. I was born this way. Why did you hurt me?" "Oh, I'm sorry," Martha said as she reached out her arms to hug Judy, "I didn't know that. Please forgive me. I want to help you. Can we be friends?"

What at first might seem to be ridicule, may not have been meant in this way. But what of course reminds one of their infirmities can cause sadness. In such a case, you might want to ask the thought provoking question: Why are you hurting me? This was the case with Judy, a sixth-grade student who used a wheelchair, when she had just been integrated into a school with able-bodied students.

Another technique a disabled individual can use when responding in such circumstances is to ask the question: "Would you like to have a disability?"

Would You Like To Have My Disability?: Bill, Paul and James walked over to Jimmy who lay reclined in his wheelchair. James snickered, "Some people have it so good. You ride around and are lazy. Do you play sports?," Jimmy asked. "Well yeah!," the boys replied. "We play baseball and football. Now, think a moment," Jimmy replied. "How would you like to have my problem and not be able to kick a ball or swing a bat?" The boys lowered their heads and walked away in shame.

This chapter has explored how to cope with the stares, taunts, ridicule and questions about your medical condition. This is often distressful because no one wants to feel unwanted, odd or unequal to others. Learning ways to cope with such situations appropriately can help develop positive self-esteem and build better interpersonal relationships.

Points To Remember

1. Understand the reason for ridicule and questions about your disability: Adults don't always know how to react, and children are curious.

2. Why children mimic physically challenged people: They don't know it is not acceptable and may wonder about the strange mannerisms of the person. Youngsters can be curious. They want to "show off" to their peers. Teenagers may decide that associating with a disabled person is embarrassing.

3. Handicapped people can be affected differently to situations: Try to react positively.

4. There are different methods of responding to questions and ridicule: When answering questions, be forthright, use simple language, explain the medical aspect, and help parents answer children's inquiries. There are ways of dealing with ridicule. Anger may not be helpful, avoid self-pity and depression, overlook taunts, deal with name calling, by asking: "Why do you hurt me? Would you like to be disabled?"

Chapter 11

You And The Able-Bodied

Frank Myer, who was born with a speech impediment, had to move. He tried phoning several moving companies, but often they hung up on him, not being able to comprehend what he was saying.

Jerry James, who walked with a limp, had volunteered at a handicapped recreational program for seven years and was refused employment when he applied for a job.

Susan Botts, confined to a wheelchair, wanted to attend a weekend service retreat, but she was told it was impossible for her to go because the committee did not want to take responsibility for her care.

It can be emotionally painful when coping with the prejudices against us. Both the feelings of victimization, or self-pity and rejection are understandable, but not helpful. Therefore, why not take a positive attitude in these situations rather than allowing them to devastate you.

View Yourself As Equal

To associate with people effectively, you should view yourself as an equal in many respects. What are some methods you can use? Here are five suggestions:

Don't Focus On Your Physical Appearance: Never become too self-conscious about your appearance, that is, as it relates to obvious impairments. For instance, if you have difficulty walking and find that it takes a great deal of energy while also causing pain, don't be embarrassed to use a wheelchair.

Know Your Own Worth: All the way through this book, I have stressed the importance of having a good self-appraisal of who you are. Why is this so important in your interpersonal relationships?

1. Should you project a low opinion of yourself, others may take a similar view. They might try consoling you for a time, but this becomes tiresome, and your associates may not continue making an effort to help after awhile.

2. If you believe that you are not on a par with those who seem unlimited, and you project that image, some may try, and often will, take advantage of you.

3. If you are a handicapped individual who has a sullen attitude, this may turn people away from maintaining the association.

Mingle With The Able-Bodied: Do you ever find it difficult to associate with those having no physical impairments? Wait a minute! Remember, that we all have insecurities. Many of us are shy. Many of us are withdrawn for various reasons. Frequently, the non-disabled find it difficult to talk with someone less fortunate. If this is the case, why not pursue the matter and break the ice. Take the chance; you might make a friend.

You Have Talents Nobody Else Has: No matter how disabled you may be—you have attributes no one else has. For example, someone asked the parents of a mentally retarded child why they did not institutionalize him. They responded, "Oh no! We could not do that! He gives us so much love!" As you will note, even the most severely afflicted person can give something to others.

You Are No Less Important: The facts are that you are not less important than anyone else. Don't let people indicate otherwise. Never buy the lie that just because you are handicapped, you must be dependent—financially, psychologically or socially. Be strong and determined that you will take a "fight back" position and project a self-assured attitude to those you meet.

We Are Vulnerable

While it is a good idea to think of ourselves as equal to others in so many ways, we must realize that we are vulnerable to victimization by unscrupulous, unethical persons. Here are a few examples:

RAPE: A high percentage of disabled people have been or will be raped. With the growing rise of pornography and sexual immorality, acts such as these are prevalent in our society today.

Other Criminal Behavior: A few years ago there was an article in a *San Francisco* newspaper about someone having taken a purse from a woman sitting in her wheelchair.

In another case, a man offered to wheel a youth in his chair. A billfold was lying in the youth's lap. The would-be helper grabbed the wallet, and the young man was left without any money.

Aviod Financial Schemes: Some unfortunate people want to be employed so badly, they fall for financial schemes. There is a certain amount of risk in every area of your life. It is fine to take chances, but try small ones, so if the venture isn't successful, then you have not lost much.

Be On Guard

It is sad to say, as just previously illustrated, people do take advantage of those who are limited. There are many reasons for this. Individuals relate to disabled people as helpless, they view them as mentally deficient, and some persons consider the handicapped as emotionally inferior.

How can you protect yourself from being one who is misjudged? Here are several procedures which could help eliminate adverse opinions of us which could occur:

Physical Helplessness: Some who are disabled have determined how to defend themselves. One physically-limited youth learned Judo as a means of protecting himself.

Another suggestion is to stay away from areas of the city where there is a high crime rate; you are especially subject to being attacked at night.

Mental Helplessness: Those of you reading this book are able to analyze things use your mental abilities to determine when mind and figure out when someone is taking advantage of you. Then don't allow the circumstance to happen.

Emotional Helplessness: You can avoid the appearance of emotional inadequacy by trying to remain on a healthy status emotionally. Learn to deal successfully with negative feelings such as anger, self-pity and depression. Admittedly, this may be difficult at times, but we all should keep working at it.

Identifying Double Talk And Lying

Often people will double-talk and lie to the limited. What is double talk? It is simply stating something when your intention is to do the opposite. In other words, deceptive talk. For example, Jerry had a friend who kept telling him that he would come to visit, but the person invariable came late or not at all. On the other hand, lying is stating something that is just false.

How do you cope with such behavior? Here are four ways:

1. Be Patient: Your first reaction should be one of patience. For example, this author has a frustrating problem with people who are late for appointments. If I am not on guard, I tend to worry, become angry and to develop a dislike for the tardy one. Here is a story about a baseball coach, whose players kept coming late for practice. One day he told them this should never happen again. The next day, the star pitcher Joey did not come. The coach was furious. Later that night, Joey phoned to apologize, but he heard a long lecture. When it was finished, he said, "Sorry coach for letting you down, but my mother died today."

So, you should understand that sometimes even the best intentioned people are unable to always keep their promises.

Confront the Person: If others repeatedly continue to lie or double-talk, confront them about the problem. For instance, on the issue of being late, if the individual constantly makes appointments with you and is generally late or never comes at all, talk to the person about the matter. You might want to explain to him that the inconvenience with this type of behavior is affecting your relationship. You could add that his actions disrupt your schedule and you think it is unnecessary. Then perhaps you might want to suggest some guidelines such as, "Be sure to phone if you are unable to keep an appointment. When I am not at home, put your message on my answering machine."

Give a Warning: If someone refuses to abide by your comments and continues in the same style, you might find it urgent to give a second warning. You may wish to say something like this, "We discussed being prompt sometime ago, but conditions have not improved. I cannot allow you to keep missing appointments without notifying me. This situation must change shortly or I will refuse any meetings in the future."

Disassociate Yourself: When a person refuses your last warning, then it is time to take action. Perhaps, he or she does not really respect you. Of course, there could be many reasons for taking such an attitude. The one whose word cannot be trusted, is not worthy of your companionship.

Coping With Disparaging Behavior

One of the best ways to describe disparaging behavior, is that many people have the "poor little you" attitude toward someone who has been injured. For the person experiencing this treatment, it can really damage self-esteem.

One Sunday after church, Mrs. Bobbs approached Don, who was sitting in his chair waiting for a bus to take him home, and said, "You poor, poor thing. I am so sorry for you." Without asking permission, she grabbed his shoulder and said, "Oh God , heal this person from his suffering, or take him into your kingdom."

Don, feeling humiliated, slapped her hand, while sharply replying, "Take your filthy hands off me!" Perhaps this was not the best response, but it is understandable that Don would feel this way.

How can a disabled person adjust to behavior that tends to lower one's self esteem? Here are some suggestions:

Ignore the Behavior: Able-bodied people may not understand how to relate to those with physical limitations. Remember, this is not your problem. It is the other person's problem. Avoid extreme negative emotions, such as anger and self-pity. As an old saying states, "just consider the source." An angry reaction only hurts you.

Make Your Best Appearance: To avoid the possibility of others feeling sorry for you and displaying a minimizing attitude in your presence, refrain from reaching out for pity. Try to leave an impression of being self-assured and in control of your life. Attempt to prove to others that you do not need their sympathy, and that you have abilities despite your limitations.

Disassociate Yourself From the Person: If you have someone in your life who takes a discrediting approach toward you and refuses to acknowledge your potential, disassociate yourself from the individual. It is difficult remaining positive while in the company of someone who is negative about your circumstances. Be wise. Remove yourself from the situation.

Dealing With Discrimination

For a disabled person, at times life seems unfair. Even though laws do exist, discrimination does occur. Why does this happen? Here are two causes; people do not understand the needs of the limited or their potential and often some non-handicapped persons lack patience, and are reluctant to give the injured one an opportunity to prove his or her abilities.

Laws of Protection: There are many laws that protect the disabled from discrimination. If you are interested in a complete overview of such regulations, you can obtain the *Summary of Existing Legislation Relating to the Handicapped.* Here are just a few examples:

Rehabilitation Act Of 1973: This act is divided into three parts. Section 504 of this Act states:

> "No otherwise qualified handicapped individual in the United States as defined in Section 7(7), shall by reason of his handicap be excluded from participation in, be denied the benefits of, or be subjected to discrimination under any program or activity conducted by any Executive agency or by the United States Postal Service.

Section 7(7) defines the term "handicapped individual" to mean: "any person who has a physical or mental impairment which substantially limits one or more of such person's major life activities; has a record of such an impairment, or is regarded as having such an impairment.

Sections 501 and 503 of the Act protects handicapped persons from employment discrimination by Federal contractors. Each Federal agency is required under Section 501 to develop an affirmative action plan for hiring, placing, and advancing handicapped individuals within the agency. An Interagency Committee of Handicapped Employees is established under Section 501 to monitor implementation of this Act.

Education Of The Handicapped: The education of the Handicapped Act, as amended, expressed Congressional intent that all handicapped children have a right to appropriate free public education. Section 3(c) of the Act states:

> "It is the purpose of this Act that all handicapped children have available to them, within the time periods specified in Section 612 (2), a free appropriate public education which emphasizes special education and related services designed to meet their unique needs, to assure that the rights of handicapped children and their parents or guardians are protected, to assist states and localities to provide for the education of all handicapped children, and to assess and assure the effectiveness of efforts to educate handicapped children."

Bill Of Rights For
The Developmentally Disabled

Section 111 of the Developmental Disabilities Assistance Bill of Rights Act, as amended, sets forth the following congressional findings respecting the rights of persons with developmental disabilities:

(1) that persons with developmental disabilities have a right to appropriate treatment, services, and habilitation, in the least restrictive settings, which are designed to maximize their developmental potential.

(2) the Federal Government and the state both have an obligation to assure that public funds are not provided to any institutional or other residential program, which does not provide treatment, services and habilitation appropriate to the needs of the developmentally disabled persons they serve; or fails to meet the following minimum standards:

* provision of a nourishing well-balanced diet.

* provision of appropriate medical and dental services.

* maintenance and enforcement of policies prohibiting the use of physical restraint unless absolutely necessary.

* maintenance and enforcement of policies prohibiting the excessive useof chemical restraints.

* policies granting permission for close relatives to visit residents at reasonable hours without prior notice.

* compliance with adequate fire and safety standards.

Think Rationally: You feel you have been discriminated against. You are angry and want to sue. Consider the following factors: A court case can take considerable time. It could be months while you are in a state of anxiety. Also, just because you were hurt emotionally, may or may not be good reason for a case. You must prove to a judge or jury that you suffered significant financial damage. It is always sensible to give yourself considerable time for intense emotions to wane before contemplating going to court.

Confronting Your Opposition: At times you may have the idea that you must confront your opposition. However, in order to do this effectively, you should use certain techniques that bring results.

1. Remember to avoid anger and think rationally about the points you wish to convey.

2. Gather any evidence which might help prove your case.

3. Be sure you know what you are going to say. Have the major points outlined in your mind.

4. Be assertive. Know your rights, and be prepared to fight for them.

Where to go For Help: If you feel you have a valid discrimination case, and are unable to fight it yourself, many resources are available. Of course, there is always the option of hiring a private lawyer, but be careful. There is a wide difference in prices as well as services. Some communities may also have low cost legal aid centers for disabled individuals.

Forgiving And Forgetting

Judy sat in her wheelchair, paralyzed and in a courtroom as the judge pronounced sixteen-year-old Steven with only a one-year sentence for drunken driving. In her mind she thought: "It is just not fair. He gets one year; I must spend my life in this chair having nurses feed and groom me. It's just not fair. It's just not fair."

Yes, at times this is true. In certain situations, people are treated poorly. On these occasions, as in the case of Judy, it means forgiving those who have caused great personal injury. So, why must we forgive? Here are four good reasons:

To Overcome Negative Emotions: Anger, bitterness, or depression can often be traced to lack of forgiveness. Certainly, this is not to say that a grievance toward you was right, when in fact it was wrong. How long are you going to allow the incident to wound you—a day, a week, a month, a year, or an entire life time? Instead of holding on to the hurt, won't it be wiser to let it go.

To Develop Healthy Interpersonal Relationships: There are people who seem to delight in living in the past. They might blame others for their misfortunes.

Such persons can drive prospective friends away. Some who will not forgive, have difficulty trusting others.

To Set New Goals: There are those who have problems with forgetting earlier troublesome experiences, so they struggle when making plans for the future. Often, one must erase the bad memories, however deeply entrenched they may be. It is quite difficult to chart a new course, perhaps even rebuilding dreams which are shattered, if there remains a thorn of unforgiveness with you that keeps gnawing away.

To Forget: Forgiving must involve forgetting. This does not indicate you will never think of the incident again, but for your own well-being you should reach a place whereby you are in control of your negative emotions. Not only is this necessary in the area of goal setting, but in every area of your life as well. It is not easy to obliterate bad memories from the mind, but you will be happier when you have learned not to be emotionally wounded each time you think of them.

It is frequently troublesome for the able-bodied to interact with physically-impaired people. Sometimes it is advantageous for the limited-person to be tactful in an effort to put the uncomfortable one at ease. Hopefully, this chapter has provided some ideas that may prove helpful.

Points To Remember

1. View Yourself as Equal: Don't focus on your appearance, relating to your physical limitations. Know your own worth. Mingle with able-bodied people. You have talents nobody else has. You are no less important..

2. Disabled People Are Vulnerable to Rape, and Various Other Forms of Criminal Behavior and Financial Schemes.

3. Be On Guard: Prevent others from treating you as helpless, mentally deficient, and emotionally impaired by doing whatever you can to better your self-image.

4. Identify Double Talk and Lying: Be patient. Confront the person. Give a warning. Disassociate yourself from those with whom you are not compatible.

5. Coping With Disparaging Behavior: Ignore other's inappropriate actions. Make your best appearance, and if you must, refrain from being in the company of those who belittle you.

6. Dealing With Discrimination: There are many laws that protect disabled people from discrimination. Think rationally; don't become "sue happy." Confront your opposition. Seek professional help.

7. Forgiving and Forgetting is Important: These steps are essential to overcome negative emotions, to develop healthy interpersonal relationships, to set new goals, and to erase unpleasant memories. Consistently strive to improve in those areas. Then, forgive and forget.

A Concluding Thought

Let's share some final thoughts and consider how to apply this material to your daily life. Realize that what has been covered could be summarized in one sentence: Accepting physical limitations involves adjusting to your disability, living with it positively and creatively, while also building good public relations with others. The proceeding pages have discussed many suggestions.

It has been said that ideas are a dime a dozen. They are worth nothing unless you apply them. However, since you have finished this book, you must have wanted to change your life to become a happier, more successful, and more productive person.

Using this guidebook, start on your journey. Believe in yourself. Don't look back. Look ahead to a bright future which awaits you and move forward anticipating success.

Order Form

Use this coupon to order additional copies of
ACCEPTING DISABILITY.

-- -- -- -- -- -- -- -- -- -- -- -- -- -- -- -- -- --

YES! Please send me _____ copies @ $12.95 each of:
ACCEPTING DISABILITY
by Hoyt Anderson

(Please add $2.00 postage and handling for one book, and 50¢
for each additional book. California residents add sales tax).

Name: _____

Address: _____

City: _____ State: _____ Zip: _____

Send to:

Disabled Resource Services
P.O. Box 163656
Sacramento, CA 95816